the **yoga back** book

the **yoga back** book

Stella Weller

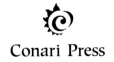

Conari Press

This edition first published by Thorsons in 1993.
A revised edition was published in 2000.

This edition published in 2012 by Conari Press,
an imprint of Red Wheel/Weiser, LLC
With offices at:
665 Third Street, Suite 400
San Francisco, CA 94107
www.redwheelweiser.com

ISBN: 978-1-57324-576-0

Photography by Robin Matthews
Text illustrations by Pete Cox Associates
Cover Design: Adrian Morgan
Cover image © Jeff Thrower

Printed and bound in China by South China Printing Co. Ltd

Contents

Acknowledgments

Many people have contributed to this revised version of *The Yoga Back Book* and I now thank them all.

I am particularly grateful to my husband, Walter, and to Samantha Grant, Assistant Health Editor at Thorsons. I also thank Lara Burgess, Lizzy Gray, Lora Galloway, Gia Bettencourt-Gomes, Diana Harland, Jacqui Caulton and Gideon Reeve.

Introduction

Back problems have become epidemic. Almost every one of us will experience some form of backache or pain, or related symptom at some stage of our life. Many of us will subject ourselves to unnecessary, ineffective treatments or give up activities we enjoy. Back problems, moreover, have become extremely costly: they result in absenteeism from work and they generate incalculable misery.

And yet according to experts, the care and management of our back is essentially *our* responsibility, and self-treatment of low back pain and similar problems brings better and more lasting results, in the long-term, than any other form of therapy.

For almost fifty years, I have lived a full and highly productive life, despite a marked lateral curvature of the spine (scoliosis). I attribute this, in large part, to the observation and practice of principles of back care which I now share with you in this book. These are based on the ancient wisdom of yoga – a system of non-strenuous exercises done with full awareness, in synchronization with appropriate breathing, and special mental and breathing exercises that promote relaxation and help in coping with stress.

Yoga, which was tremendously popular in the 1960s and 1970s is now making a strong comeback. I believe this is because of people's disenchantment with the unfulfilled promises of many high-impact, aerobic-type exercises and the potential of some of them for injury. Yoga is ideal for the millions of people who suffer from backache and related problems. Its gentle movements and the concentration and synchronized breathing it requires make it impossible to hurt yourself, provided the rules are adhered to. One eminent orthopaedic specialist has written, in fact, that as controlled stretching exercise yoga has no peer, and that the mental and physical discipline involved in its practice is superb. Other authors of books on back care have devoted entire chapters to exercises to which they refer as 'similar to yoga', an acknowledgement of the respect with which the yoga system is regarded.

This book is intended not only for those of you who are plagued with back problems, but also for those of the privileged minority who aren't and who wish to keep it that way. It can also be a useful reference for health care professionals such as doctors, nurses, physiotherapists and fitness instructors. It emphasizes personal responsibility in the management of back problems. It also stresses prevention, and provides the tools to help forestall difficulties and maintain the health of the spine and related structures. These tools include information on how the vertebral (spinal) column is constructed, how to use it intelligently and how to care for it through a sensible balance of appropriate exercises, relaxation and sound nutrition.

More than 130 illustrations and photographs complement clear instructions for performing the exercises correctly and safely. These include not only back exercises but also exercises for the legs and abdomen, which are crucial to the health of the back. An entire chapter has been devoted to the principles of good body mechanics, knowledge of which is vital to the prevention of back injury. Yet another chapter focuses on the special needs of those with problems such as chronic fatigue and difficulty with sex, while useful direction is given to pre- and post-natal women.

Hippocrates, known as the father of medicine, emphasized prevention and an awareness of the whole person when treating illness. An important part of this emphasis was the education and encouragement of patients to take responsibility in assisting the therapist with their own care. *The Yoga Back Book* does just that, and provides information and instruction for helping to put those principles into safe, pleasurable practice in order to bring about the desired results.

Before driving a car or using a piece of machinery, people usually acquaint themselves with the way it works. This allows them to operate it intelligently and therefore safely. The human spine, which is perhaps more sophisticated in its design than most machines, should be similarly considered.

A basic understanding of how the spine is constructed and how it functions is therefore a vital first step towards acquiring and maintaining a trouble-free back. This chapter represents that important first step. Spend a few minutes reading it from beginning to end. The time you invest in doing so will be rewarded; it will equip you to care for your back with insight and wisdom.

Functions and Structure

The spine supports the head and about 90 per cent of the weight of the human body in an upright position. It is mechanically balanced to conform to the stress of gravity and to permit movement from place to place, as well as to assist in purposeful movements.

The spine prevents shock to the brain and spinal cord during activities (such as running and jumping) through its curves and intervertebral discs, about which more information will be given later. It protects and houses the spinal cord. It provides attachment for many powerful muscles and it forms a strong posterior boundary for the body.

Known also as the spinal or vertebral column, the spine is composed of 33 bones (vertebrae; singular, vertebra) with a pad of cartilage, or gristle (intervertebral disc) in between every two bones (Fig. 1, Fig. 2 and Fig. 3). This disc buffers the vertebrae against shock during activities such as running, jumping or driving on bumpy roads.

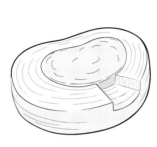 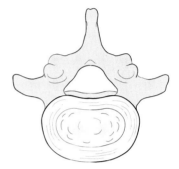

Fig.1. Intervertebral disc

The Discs

The disc has a tough elastic shell composed of crisscrossing fibres. Inside it (the nucleus) is a soft substance with the consistency of jelly. The upper and lower surfaces of the disc have a cartilaginous layer known as an end plate. This acts somewhat like a sieve between the disc and the bone.

Discs have no blood supply; they depend on a process of diffusion through the end plates for their nutrition. When we are resting or sleeping, the discs suck in water and other nutrients. When we move about or exercise, compression squeezes fluids out and expels wastes. A sensible balance of exercise and rest is therefore crucial in maintaining the health of the intervertebral discs.

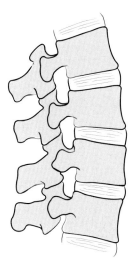

Fig. 2. Vertebrae with intervening discs

All individuals can expect degenerative changes in the discs. Between the ages of 20 and 30, maximum development of the discs has occurred and the water content is maximal – about 80 per cent. This lessens with age. With a healthy lifestyle, however, it is possible to keep the discs from drying out, and to preserve a good balance between fibre and fluid, even into advanced age.

Spinal Units

You may also think of the spine as being composed of a number of functional units. Each unit (Fig. 2) consists of two segments: an anterior (front) portion which may be considered a hydraulic, weight-bearing, shock-absorbing structure comprising two vertebrae with a disc in between them, and a posterior (back) portion which may be thought of as a guiding mechanism. This includes three projecting pieces of bone: two projecting sideways and one rearward. You may be able to feel these as 'buttons' down the middle of your back. These processes provide for the attachment of ligaments and muscles.

In addition, the rear portion of the vertebra has two upper and two lower surfaces called facets. The lower facets of one vertebra glide along those of the vertebra below. The facets thus guide and limit the motion of one vertebra relative to its neighbouring vertebra.

The articulated posterior processes of the vertebrae form a canal which houses and protects the spinal cord. This is a bundle of nerve fibres connecting the brain with all parts of the body, and which carries messages to and from the brain.

On each side of the spine, between every two vertebrae, are tiny openings for the passage of nerves branching from the spinal cord.

Ligaments and Muscles

Strengthening the joints formed by the vertebrae and their intervening discs are ligaments – tough fibrous bands of tissue – running behind and in front of them along the entire length of the spine.

Reinforcement is also provided by the back muscles which help to control forward bending, and indirectly by the abdominal ('tummy') muscles which give a counterbalancing effect and help to prevent extreme backward bending.

It is worth noting that although the abdominal muscles are not directly attached to the spine, their strength and tone are crucial to the overall health of the back.

Connective Tissue

The space between the bones, tendons, ligaments and muscles of the back are filled with material known as connective tissue. Much of this filling is composed of a protein substance known as *collagen*. In fact, collagen accounts for about 30 per cent of total body protein. It is a sort of 'cement', which binds cells together. It is the key to the relationship between nutrition and spinal health. It acts as a transport medium, carrying nutrients from the bloodstream to the muscles and ligaments, and conveying wastes to the bowel and skin for elimination.

The chief functions of connective tissue in the back are: to bind tendons to bones and buffer muscles and ligaments to help to maintain resilience and strength; and to act as a medium of transport carrying oxygen and nutrients to spinal structures and removing wastes.

Spinal Curves

With your mind's eye now, try to see the spinal column from the side (laterally). You will note four curves (Fig. 3): in the neck (cervical) region, one that is convex towards the front (lordosis); in the chest (thoracic) area, one that is convex towards the rear (kyphosis); at waist level (lumbar spine) another arch that is convex towards the front, and at hip level (sacral area) another arch that is convex towards the rear. These curves transect the plumb line of gravity in order to maintain a state of balance.

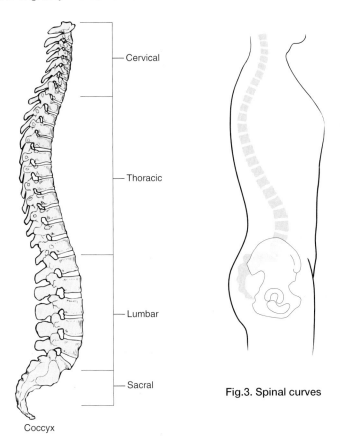

Cervical

Thoracic

Lumbar

Sacral

Coccyx

Fig.3. Spinal curves

The Pelvic Ring

The spine is balanced on an undulating pelvic base known as the pelvic ring (sometimes pelvic girdle). (Fig 4.). This is the human body's chief weight-transmitting structure, connecting the upper body to the legs. It consists of the *sacrum* at the back, and two *innominate* (hip) *bones* which are connected to the *femurs* (thigh bones). Together, these bones form five joints: two *sacroiliac* joints at the base of the spine; two hip joints where the hip bones connect with the legs, and the *symphyis pubis* where the two hip bones join in front.

A key feature of the pelvic ring is its strong ligamentous support, which is especially important in weight bearing.

During normal standing or sitting, the ligaments of the sacroiliac joints and the pelvic ring are somewhat loose. When weight bearing occurs, however, the pressure exerted down through the spinal column causes the sacroiliac ligaments to tighten. This tightening alters the position of the pelvic ring from a loose, or neutral structure to one that makes for greater stability.

A second key characteristic of the pelvic ring is that its degree of tilt determines the quality of the curves in the spinal column above. Any change in the angle of the sacral portion of the pelvis will influence the curves of the spine above, thus determining posture. If the pelvic ring is in a balanced position, the spinal curves will be proportionately balanced and the

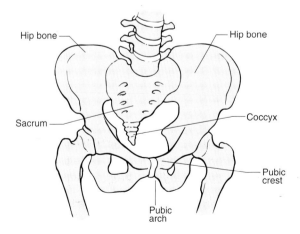

Hip bone

Hip bone

Sacrum

Coccyx

Pubic crest

Pubic arch

Fig. 4. The pelvic ring

posture safe. If, however, the pelvic ring is abnormally tilted, poor posture will result and the spine will consequently be more vulnerable to injury and pain.

Good posture and smooth movement and rhythm require good coordination between nerves and muscles, good flexibility of tissues and adequate functioning of all joints involved.

Muscular Supports

The chief back muscles are as follows:

The *erector spinae* muscles form two columns, one on each side of the spine. They extend the spine and keep the trunk erect.

The *latissimus dorsi* is a broad, flat muscle lying over the lower part of the chest and loins (between ribs and hip bones). It draws the upper bone of the arm (humerus) down and back, and rotates the arm inwards.

The *gluteal muscles*, which form the buttocks, raise the trunk from a stooping to an erect position. They are also involved in leg motions.

The *sling muscles* (hip flexors) connect the transverse processes of the spine on the inside (the projecting pieces of bone mentioned in the section 'Spinal Units'), cross the pelvic ring and attach to the thigh bones just below the hips. They are very important in the maintenance of upright posture.

The *lateral muscles* are situated between the ribcage and the pelvic ring. They extend from the lowest ribs to the hip area and legs.

Secondary Supports

Muscles forming secondary supports to the spine are: the *quadriceps* (thigh muscles), which run down the front of the thighs and insert into the kneecaps or patellae, and serve to extend the knees; and the *hamstrings*, which are located at the back of the thighs, passing from the pelvic ring and inserting into the bones of the lower legs (tibiae and fibulae). The hamstrings flex the knees and extend the thighs.

Both sets of muscles – quadriceps and hamstrings – contribute to the tilt or balance of the pelvic ring and so are important to good posture.

The abdominal muscles, which will be dealt with in chapter six, basically extend from the breastbone (sternum) to the symphysis pubis, on each side of the midline. Although thin, these muscles give extremely important support to the spine. They operate at a distance and so provide leverage.

Postural patterns are influenced not only by lifestyle but also by genetic and early environmental factors. Without conscious, sustained effort, faulty postures can become permanent.

There is no ideal posture, since people come in all shapes and sizes. The ideal posture for you is one in which your back is subjected to the least possible strain and in which the normal graceful curves of the spine are maintained.

The key to good posture is fitness. If you keep your muscles well conditioned, you stand a good chance of acquiring the posture that is correct for you, particularly if you complement this with a balanced mental and emotional state. This is the essence of the yoga approach.

Dr Bess Mensendieck, a sculptor turned physician, has remarked that correct posture, and freedom from pain due to faulty posture, can be acquired only when all muscles are used in accordance with their anatomical functions and with the laws of body mechanics. She has further noted that the primary exercise needed to achieve these states is the practice of correct postural habits during normal daily activities. No daily half-hour exercise session alone will produce good posture if muscles and joints and related structures are not used properly the rest of the time.

A well-aligned vertebral column when we are upright or sit or lie down imposes the least strain on the spine. It is also an important prerequisite for the harmonious functioning of the nervous system, which is hinged on the backbone and the spinal cord, and for the free expansion of the chest to permit proper breathing. If we can maintain natural physical equilibrium when both sitting and standing, we minimize strain on the back muscles and facilitate harmonious distribution of the body weight along the 132 articulations of the vertebral column.

In summary, your posture is determined by the way you hold each part of your body, from head to toes. Your posture affects your breathing, indeed your health in general – both physical and emotional – and the image your present to the world.

In order to relieve stress on the lumbar spine, a natural lumbar curvature (at the small of the back), good balance and flexibility must be maintained at all times. The natural lumbar curvature is maintained through pelvic tilt (assisted by tightening abdominal and buttock muscles). The position distributes weight evenly down through the spine allowing the strong leg muscles to bear the weight.

Now that you have a basic understanding of the structure and function of the spine, you will readily appreciate the principles of good body mechanics which follow and the importance of maintaining the normal spinal curves.

Sitting

Good posture when sitting puts the pelvis in a neutral position, that is, neither tilted backwards not tilted forwards (remember that posture is controlled mainly from the pelvis).

The spine should be supported along its natural curve. The height of the seat should be such as to place the knees level with, or higher than, the hips (Fig. 5).

Figures 6 and 7 are examples of poor posture in sitting. In Fig. 6 the pelvis is tilted backwards. This flattens the normal curve of the lower spine, stretching ligaments and eventually producing pain.

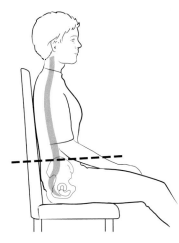

Fig. 5. Good posture in sitting

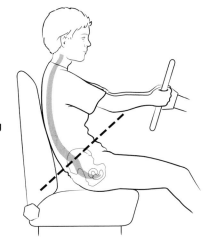

Fig. 6. Poor posture in sitting

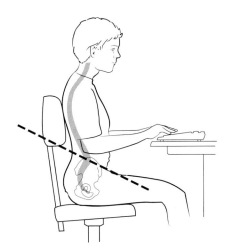

Fig. 7. Poor posture in sitting

In Fig. 7 the pelvis is tilted forwards, thus distorting good posture in much the same way as prolonged standing does. This, too, can lead to back strain and pain.

The Easy Pose

One excellent way to sit is in the yoga *Easy Pose* (Fig. 8). It provides a stable base, encourages you to hold your spine naturally erect and promotes relaxation of the back muscles. It brings into play the sartorius, or tailor, muscles which lie across the thighs, from about the front of the hip bones to what we know as the shin bones. These are the muscles used in bending the legs and turning them inwards.

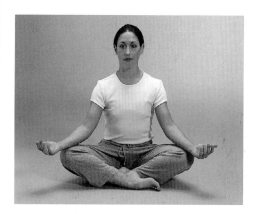

Fig. 8. Easy Pose

Here's how to do the *Easy Pose*.

1　Sit with your legs stretched out in front.
2　Bend one leg and place the foot under the opposite thigh.
3　Bend the other leg and place the foot under the other bent leg.
4　Rest your palms quietly on the respective knees or place them upturned, one in the other, in your lap.
5　Maintain this posture as long as you comfortably can, breathing regularly, and keeping your body relaxed.

Note

If your knees do not touch the surface on which you are sitting, do not be discouraged. They eventually will as your joints become more flexible and your ligaments more elastic.

The Japanese Sitting Position

Here's another position that encourages good posture in sitting (Fig. 9).

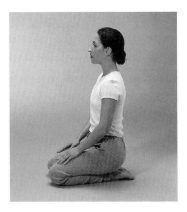

Fig. 9. Japanese Sitting Position

1   Kneel down with your legs together and your body erect but not rigid. Let your feet point straight backwards.
2   Slowly lower your body to sit on your heels. Rest your palms quietly on the respective knees. Sit tall and breathe regularly. Keep as relaxed as you can.

Note

If at first your heels cannot bear your weight, place a cushion between your bottom and heels, and hold the position only briefly. As your knees and ankles become more flexible and your body more conditioned, you will be able to sit in this posture for a longer time.

Squatting

One quarter of the human race habitually take weight off its feet by squatting. A deep squat position for work and rest is used by millions of people in Africa, Asia and Latin America.

Squatting reduces any exaggerated curve of the lower spine, thus lessening tension in spinal muscles and ligaments. It reduces pressure on the spinal discs. As a result, the back is both strengthened and relaxed, and back discomforts are minimized. Squatting is, moreover, excellent for strengthening the ankles and feet.

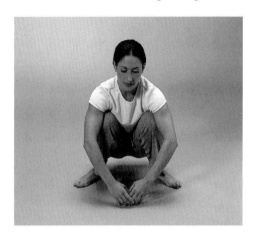

Fig. 10. Squatting

The Squatting Pose

1   Stand with your legs comfortably apart. Distribute your body weight equally between your feet. Breathe regularly.
2   Slowly bend your knees, lowering your bottom until you are sitting on your heels. Relax your arms for maximum comfort (Fig. 10). Hold this posture as long as you can, breathing regularly.
3   Resume your starting position. Rest.

Note well

If you have varicose veins, you would do better to practise the dynamic version of the Squatting Pose which follows, rather than holding the squat for any length of time.

The Squatting Pose – Dynamic version

1   Stand with legs apart and arms at your sides. Inhale and slowly raise your arms to shoulder level as you simultaneously raise yourself on your toes. (If you have difficulty keeping your balance, use a stable prop for support.)
2   Exhale and slowly lower your arms as you lower your body into the squatting posture (Fig. 10).
3   Without holding the posture, come up again on tiptoe. Repeat the up-and-down movements in smooth succession as many times as you wish. Relax afterwards.

This version of the Squatting Pose gives a gentle, therapeutic massage to the legs and stimulates the blood circulation.

Sitting to Prevent Backache

- Sitting puts great pressure on spinal discs. Take periodic breaks from prolonged sitting to practise stretching and relaxation exercises. Two examples will be given later in this chapter.
- Be sure that the seat on which you habitually sit to do your work is well designed. It should be fully adjustable to suit your own measurements. It should support your back and legs comfortably. It should be at a height that permits you to do your work without having to stretch your arms forwards from the shoulders. It should be adequately padded yet firm. You might consider using a desk or other work surface that slopes towards you, so that you don't have to bend your head and neck down.
- **Do** arrange things on your desk so as to avoid having to twist back and forth.
- **Don't** cradle the telephone between your ear and shoulder. It promotes upper back tension.

- **Do** rest your arms on armrests when they're available.
- **Do** consider using a lumbar roll (back log), which is a support specially designed for the low back. Use it to good advantage when reading, writing, watching television or driving your car to counteract any tendency to slouch. An ordinary cushion is not to be relied upon for long-term use; only in an emergency.

Back Break

To relieve back tension which builds up during prolonged sitting, a 'back break' is ideal. Get up from your seat and practise exercises to counteract the forward-bending attitude inherent in most sedentary activities.

Practise neck and shoulder exercises such as described in chapter four. Also practise a standing version of the *Stick Posture* (also chapter four, page 64), which is an excellent all-body stretch.

In addition, practise the two exercises to follow. Modify them to suit your needs or circumstances.

Posture Clasp

1 Sit on your heels in the *Japanese Sitting Position* (*see* Fig. 9). Breathe regularly.
2 Reach over your *right* shoulder with your *right* hand. Keep your elbow pointing upwards rather than forwards, and your arm close to your ear.
3 With your left hand, reach behind your back, from below, and interlock the fingers with those of the right hand. Maintain a naturally erect posture throughout the exercise and keep breathing (Fig. 11).
4 Hold this posture as long as you comfortably can. Do *not* hold your breath.
5 Resume your beginning position. Relax. Shrug your shoulders a few times, or rotate them, as you wish,
6 Repeat the exercise, changing the position of the arms and hands, so that the left elbow now points upwards.

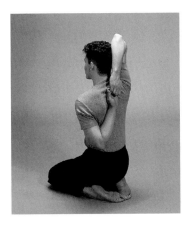

Fig. 11. Posture Clasp

Variations

- You can practise the Posture Clasp in a standing position, or sitting on a stool or bench, or in a folded-leg posture.
- If your hands don't touch each other, use a scarf or other suitable item as an extension: toss one end over your shoulder, and reach behind and below to grasp the other end. Pull upwards with the upper hand and downwards with the lower.

Chest Expander

1   Stand tall with your feet comfortably apart and your arms at your sides. Breathe regularly.
2   Inhale and raise your arms sideways to shoulder level; turn your palms downwards.
3   Exhale and lower your arms. Swing them behind you and interlace the fingers of one hand with those of the other. Maintain a naturally erect posture and keep breathing regularly.
4   With fingers still interlaced, raise your arms upwards to their comfortable limit; keep them straight (Fig. 12). Remember to maintain an erect standing position and to keep breathing regularly.

5   Hold this posture as long as you can with absolute comfort. Do **not** hold your breath.

6   Slowly lower your arms, unlock your fingers and relax. You may shrug or rotate your shoulders a few times.

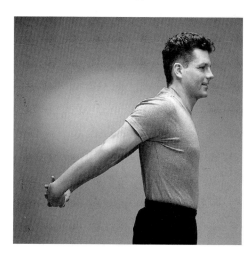

Fig. 12. Chest Expander

Variations

- Practise the Chest Expander in any comfortable sitting position.
- After completing the basic Chest Expander, slowly bend forwards, keeping your back straight and bending at your hip joints rather than at your waist. Keep your arms pushed upwards. Relax your neck. Hold the forwards bend briefly, then slowly and carefully return to your starting position. Relax. (Did you remember to keep breathing regularly?)

Standing

When we talk of poor posture, we generally mean slack posture. To correct this, there may be a tendency to cultivate posture that is excessively rigid, and this could result in tense muscles and restricted breathing.

In correct standing, the chin is in, the head up (crown uppermost), the back flattened and the pelvis straight (neutral position). The ribcage is full and round to permit adequate ventilation of the lungs and to prevent pressure on internal organs (Fig. 13).

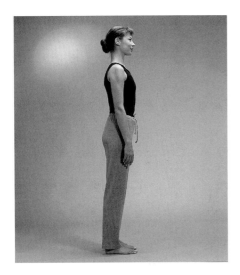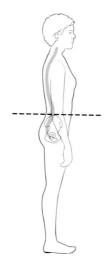

Fig. 13. Good posture in standing

In a strained position (Fig. 14), the pelvis tilts forwards, thus increasing the spinal curves and strain on joints and ligaments. The chin is out and the ribs are down, causing pressure on internal organs. The lower back is arched (swayback). This is the most common type of poor posture in a standing position.

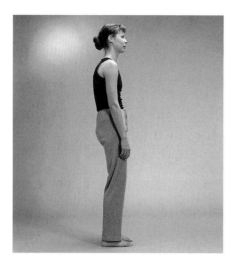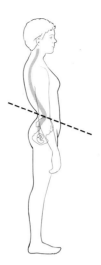

Fig. 14. Poor posture in standing

Even when standing correctly, there is tremendous pressure on lumbar discs – about 182 pounds per square inch on the third lumbar disc. Avoid standing, therefore, if you can sit, walk or squat. When you must stand, rest one foot on a convenient prop such as a bar rail, a box, a low stool or a shelf under a counter.

Walking

Stand tall to reduce stress. Relax your shoulders. Flatten your shoulderblades. Tighten your abdominal and buttock muscles to help to tuck your bottom in. Distribute your body weight equally between your feet. Breathe regularly. Swing your arms effortlessly. Move your legs from your hip joints. Practise *Diaphragmatic breathing* (*see* chapter eight, page 140) for part of your walk.

When walking up stairs, try this: Plant the whole foot on the stair instead of walking on tiptoe. It will exercise your ankle and help to conserve energy as you reach the top of the stairs.

Lying

When you lie down, you relieve your spine of much of your body weight. This reduces compression on the discs. Experiment with lying positions to find those that are most restful for you.

Lie either on your back (supine) or on your side. Avoid lying on your abdomen (prone), as it places unnecessary strain on your lower spine. When you do have to lie prone, however, place a small pillow or cushion under your hips. It will prevent exaggeration of the spinal arch and reduce tension of the back muscles.

In the supine position, you can bend your knees and rest the soles of your feet flat on the surface on which you are lying. You may experiment with inserting a large cushion, pillow or bolster under the bent knees (Fig. 15). This is a very relaxing position for the back – one recommended by many orthopaedic specialists.

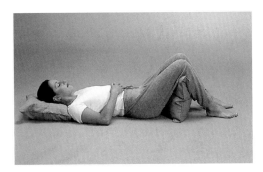

Fig. 15. Good posture in lying

I sometimes lie in a similar position, but with my knees together and bent, soles flat on the mat or sofa or bed, and feet about the hip-width apart. I find this easier to maintain for a longer time than if the knees were apart.

To counteract neck strain resulting from too much looking downwards, try rolling a towel, like a sausage, and putting it under your neck as you lie on your back for half-an-hour or so. You may also arrange the rolled towel like a collar to prevent your head from rolling to the side.

Consider using a feather or kapok pillow, which moulds itself to the contour of the head and neck while giving support and promoting relaxation. A foam pillow, by contrast, has recoil which tends to produce a certain amount of neck tension.

Your mattress should be firm yet able to conform to your body's contours without sagging.

When lying on your side, place a small pillow or cushion between your knees to prevent your hips from rotating and your spine from twisting. Both legs, or only the top one, may be bent for maximum comfort (Fig. 16).

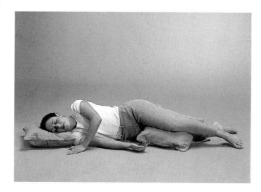

Fig. 16. Good posture in lying

Getting up (From Lying)

Never get up in a rush. Avoid getting straight upwards from a supine position. Instead, roll onto your side, bend your knees, bring them closer to your chest and use your hands to help push you onto your hip (Fig. 17).

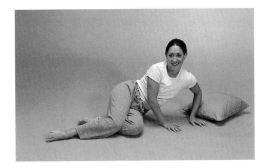

Fig. 17. Getting up safely

Slowly pivot yourself until you are sitting evenly on your bottom, then slowly stand up. Breathe regularly all the while, to help you to concentrate on what you are doing.

Carrying

To carry anything heavy – groceries for example – divide them into two parts of roughly equal weight and carry one part on each side. Alternatively, look for someone to help you or use a trolley or cart if one is available.

Use luggage trolleys or wheels, or cases with wheels when you travel. Carry a small suitcase in each hand rather than struggle with a single large suitcase. Push trolleys rather than pull them to prevent back strain.

Maintain good posture at all times and check that you are *not* holding your breath. Remember to keep breathing regularly.

Bending and Lifting

Improper bending and reassuming a standing position is one of the most frequent causes of low back pain.

You can protect your spine when lifting by holding the object close to you with both hands to prevent the body from being pulled into the poor forward-leaning posture and also to prevent twisting. Good balance and flexibility are maintained by placing the feet in a broad-based stance and by bending the knees. This stance allows the body to move as a unit, and the weight to be shifted from one leg to the other.

To avoid subjecting your back to unnecessary stress and to prevent injury, observe the following basic steps when bending and lifting:

1 Keep your back straight but not necessarily vertical. Bend your legs and lower yourself as if to squat.
2 For best balance, position your feet about shoulder-width apart, with one in front of the other. The forward foot should be flat and the rear on tiptoe, as it were. Your knee should not touch the floor (Fig. 18).
3 Securely grasp the object to be lifted. Bring it close to you. Keep your arms close to your body.
4 Get up slowly and with awareness, letting the powerful leg muscles work for you. Observe good posture. Breathe regularly.

Avoiding pitfalls

Here are more tips to help to prevent back injury when you bend and lift:

- Prepare the setting and the equipment. Render your work area safe by removing clutter, or by noting any unevenness or slipperiness of terrain, for example. Make sure there is adequate space in which to move.
- Wear suitable clothing which permits ease of movement, and which won't get caught or cause other impediment.

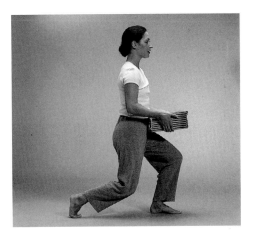 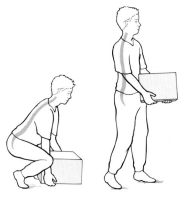

Fig. 18. Good posture in bending

- Prepare your posture: place your feet apart in a walking stance. Bend your knees. Tighten your abdominal muscles. Maintain the neutral pelvic tilt (*see* Fig. 13). Use both hands. Hold the object close to you.
- Before lifting an object, be sure that you have a secure grip on it; use aids if necessary, such as slings, ropes or a mechanical lift.
- Concentrate on what you are doing (*see* chapter eight for concentration exercises, page 137 to 138). Breathe regularly.

Reaching

Avoid back strain through overreaching. To get something from a high shelf, stand on a stable stepladder or sturdy piece of furniture so you can reach the object with ease. If you feel insecure, hold on to something safe with one hand.

Concentrate when stepping up and stepping down. Breathing regularly will help you to focus attention on what you are doing.

Vacuuming, Mopping, Shovelling, etc.

If your equipment is sufficiently lightweight, try using a lunging technique (Fig. 19) which will exercise the joints and muscles of your hips and legs. These, remember, are secondary back supports (*see* chapter one, page 7) which contribute to the health of the spine.

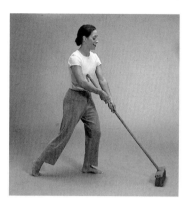

Fig. 19. Lunging

Remember to keep the back naturally straight and to breathe regularly.

If you're shovelling earth or snow, face the area you're going to dig and point the forward foot in that direction. Keep your arms close to your body. Point the rear foot towards the place where the shovelful is to be deposited and turn from the hip (rather than the waist) towards the rear foot. (Fig. 20).

Catching

Try to avoid catching falling objects. Your muscles need time to contract sufficiently to protect spinal joints, ligaments and discs. If they have to contract suddenly, without ample warning, they may not be able to co-ordinate adequately and the force involved in catching may be enough to cause damage. You may also slip and fall.

In Summary

Whether you sit, stand or walk, lie down or get up, bend, reach, lift or carry, the key to good posture is maintaining the normal curves of the spine. Any position, gesture, action or movement that alters these curves has the potential to place strain on spinal structures, weaken them, produce discomfort or pain and make the back more vulnerable to injury.

In order to maintain normal spinal curves you need to keep your back, abdominal and leg muscles in good tone and you need to guard against overweight. You also need to balance regular exercise with rest and relaxation.

It is not only sedentary workers who require exercise. Even those whose occupations involve physical labour may be using certain muscles habitually to the neglect of others. Suitable exercises, done regularly, will help to stretch out shortened muscles which contribute to poor posture. Exercise will help to keep joints freely moving and less liable to be injured. Examples of such exercises are given throughout this book.

Please remember to *check with your doctor* before practising these or any other exercises. Ask if they are suitable for *you* and compatible with treatment you may be receiving.

To stay alive and to function optimally, all living tissue needs oxygen and nutrients. The circulation through which these vital substances are delivered to the tissues must also be healthy. If the blood supply is reduced because of muscle spasm or poor posture, for example, then the nutrition to the affected parts of the body will be diminished and their function will be impaired.

It is essentially what we eat that provides the body with the raw materials for building and maintaining a healthy spine, spinal discs, muscles, connective tissues and other components of the system. Nutrients from an adequate, wholesome diet are processed by the digestive system and transported to all cells and tissues through the blood circulation.

This chapter does not offer yet another fad diet. It simply highlights nutrients that are crucial to the structure and function of the spine and its attachments. It suggests sources from which to obtain these nutrients, and alerts you to substances that work against them. Although I have focused on only a few, it is well to remember that *all* nutrients work together and that no single one can be considered a panacea.

If you are considering taking nutritional supplements, it would be prudent to consult a dietician, nutritionist or other qualified health professional first.

Vitamins

Vitamin A

This fat-soluble vitamin has a scavenging effect on *free radicals*, substances that are by-products of protein, carbohydrate and fat metabolism. They are considered 'mischievous molecules' which play a part in ageing and in cancer development. As such, vitamin A is a highly protective nutrient.

Vitamin A promotes the growth of strong bones and protects the lining of joints against inflammation. It also enhances the repair of bones and connective tissue.

Vitamin A increases the permeability of blood capillaries (small blood vessels) which carry oxygen and other vital nutrients to the body's cells. (Capillary permeability exists when the capillary wall allows blood to pass readily into cells and tissue spaces and vice versa. The more permeable the capillary walls are, the better is the supply of oxygen delivered to cells.)

In addition, vitamin A, combined with vitamin E, promotes cell oxygenation, whereby cells are supplied with oxygen.

The best sources of vitamin A include: fresh vegetables, especially intensely green and yellow ones such as broccoli, carrots, dandelion leaves, kale, parsley, spinach, squash, sweet potatoes and turnip tops, and fresh fruits such as apricots, cantaloupe melons, cherries, mangoes, papaya and peaches. Vitamin A is also obtainable from milk, milk products and fish liver oils.

The B vitamins

Called 'the nerve vitamins', this complex consists of more than twenty vitamins which are essential for maintaining a healthy nervous system and for counteracting the harmful effects of stress. The B vitamins affect the immune system, which protects us from infection and other forms of disease.

All the vitamins work together and are best obtained as a complex. They include thiamin (B_1), riboflavin (B_2), niacin (B_3), pyridoxine (B_6) – which helps to strengthen collagen and increase resistance to pain – folic acid (B_9) – which acts as an analgesic (pain reliever) – and cyanocobalamin (B_{12}).

The B vitamins may be obtained from brewer's yeast, eggs, fresh fruits, green leafy vegetables, liver, milk, nuts, pulses (dried peas, beans and lentils), seeds, wheat germ and whole grains and cereals. They are also synthesized (changed into usable form) by intestinal bacteria.

Vitamin C

This water-soluble vitamin is needed for healthy tissues, to promote healing and to reinforce resistance to disease. It must be supplied daily since it is not stored in the body.

Vitamin C is essential for the formation and maintenance of collagen, the strong cement-like material that holds cells together. As pointed out in chapter one (page 4), much of the protective connective tissue in the back is composed of collagen, which is formed largely of protein. Connective tissue plays an important role in the transport of nutrients to various structures (such as bones, tendons and muscles) and in the elimination of waste matter from them.

Vitamin C also contributes to the utilization of oxygen and to the maintenance of a healthy blood circulation. It is, in addition, an anti-stress vitamin and, like vitamins A and E, an antioxidant which helps to slow down the destructive effects of oxygen and other substances.

The best sources of vitamin C include: fresh fruits such as apricots, blackberries, cantaloupe melons, cherries, elderberries, gooseberries, grapefruit, guavas, honeydew melons, kiwi fruit, kumquats, lemons, limes, oranges, papayas, rosehips (the seed-pods of wild roses), strawberries and tangerines; fresh vegetables such as cabbage, dandelion leaves, green and red peppers, kohlrabi, mustard and cress and turnip tops.

Vitamin D

This nutrient is needed to help in absorbing the mineral calcium from the small intestine. It is also required for the assimilation of the mineral phosphorus. The action of sunlight on the skin's oils promotes its formation, and it is then absorbed through the skin back into the body. Significant reserves of vitamin D are stored in the liver, spleen, brain and bones.

Probably the most reliable source of this nutrient is vitamin D-enriched milk. Other sources include: butter, eggs, fatty fish (such as mackerel and salmon, with the skin) and fish liver oils.

Some plant foods and green leafy vegetables contain vitamin D presurcors (substances preceding other substances) known as ergosterols. Of these, parsley is a particularly rich source.

Vitamin E

Considered an anti-stress nutrient, vitamin E is also an antioxidant. In addition, it has pain-relieving properties and it helps to improve circulation.

Vitamin E plays an important role in the absorption and storage of vitamin A and it protects against environmental influences, such as radiation, which can destroy certain nutrients.

Good vitamin E sources include: almonds and other nuts (preferably eaten fresh from the shell), broccoli, Brussels sprouts, eggs, fresh fruits, green leafy vegetables, pulses, seeds, unrefined vegetable oils, wheat germ and whole grains.

Vitamin K

Known as 'the blood vitamin', this nutrient promotes proper blood clotting and so helps to prevent excessive bleeding. It is also needed for the production of the protein matrix upon which calcium is deposited to form bone. (A matrix is the basic substance from which something develops or is made.)

In addition, vitamin K is necessary for the production of osteocalcin, which helps calcium to crystallize in the bones, and speeds up the healing of fractures by stimulating bone growth. It is also of value in preventing osteoporosis.

A varied, wholesome diet usually provides enough vitamin K for normal requirements. Rich food sources include: alfalfa sprouts, cow's milk, egg yolk, fish liver oils, green leafy vegetables and kelp (a type of seaweed). Other vitamin K sources are sunflower, soya bean and other unrefined vegetable oils.

Vitamin K is also synthesized in the intestine by friendly bacteria.

Minerals

Boron

Boron helps to safeguard calcium in the body. It also appears necessary for activating vitamin D and certain hormones, such as oestrogen, which is important in preventing bone loss in women as they age.

The safest way to increase your intake of this mineral is to include boron-rich foods in your diet. These include: fresh fruits and vegetables such as alfalfa sprouts, cabbage, lettuce, peas, snap beans, apples and grapes. Other sources of boron are: almonds, dates, dried fruits, hazelnuts, peanuts, prunes, raisins, and soya beans.

Calcium

Calcium is the dominant element in human bone. The body of a healthy adult contains about three pounds of calcium (1.4 kilogrammes).

Every day you lose calcium in your urine and faeces. If you do not replace what you lose, your bones will suffer in time.

Calcium is also essential for good tone and action of the skeletal muscles (those covering the body's bony framework). It is also required for the proper functioning of nervous tissue and for normal blood clotting.

Calcium is known to relieve muscle cramps and also to promote sound sleep, which many sufferers of backache find elusive.

The best food sources of calcium include: blackstrap molasses, carob powder, citrus fruits, dried beans, dried figs, fish, green leafy vegetables (such as bok choy and spring greens, or collards), milk and milk products, peanuts, sardines, sesame seeds, soya beans and by-products such as tofu (soya bean curd), sunflower seeds, walnuts and watercress.

Milk and milk products

From the standpoint of bone health, milk has several points in its favour:

- it usually contains vitamin D, which helps the body to absorb calcium;
- it has the ideal two-to-one balance of calcium and phosphorus;
- it is a rich source of lactase, the enzyme that is needed to digest milk sugar.

If you are concerned about your fat intake, your best choices of milk are: fluid skimmed or low-fat milk; reconstituted non-fat milk powder; evaporated skimmed or low-fat milk, skimmed milk yoghurt, and buttermilk (unless you are on a low-salt diet).

Lactose intolerance

Some people cannot tolerate milk, cheese and other dairy foods because of lactose (milk sugar) intolerance. For these individuals, there are certain products on the market, such as LactAid, which, when added to milk, break down the lactose, making the milk acceptable to the digestive system.

Supplements

Calcium supplements, available at chemists and health food stores, may be a partial answer for those who are not taking in adequate amounts of this mineral through their diet. These supplements include: calcium carbonate products, calcium lactate and calcium gluconate.

Please check with your doctor or nutritionist for advice on *your* best choice of calcium supplement. Boosting calcium intake:

- Try figs for snacks. One fig contains about 23 milligrams of calcium. (Figs, however, are high in calories.)
- Sprinkle grated Parmesan cheese or toasted almonds (ground or slivered) on stir-fried broccoli.
- Use yoghurt as a base for dips, spreads and toppings.
- Try tofu in lasagne and stir-fried dishes.
- Add almonds or cheese cubes to salads.
- Use milk instead of 'whiteners' in tea and coffee.

High-calcium shake

Here's a recipe for a drink that is rich in calcium, vitamin D, silica, fluorine and other bone-strengthening nutrients. It's easy to make and it's enough for one person.

Into an electric blender (or equivalent), pour a cup of chilled, low-fat, vitamin D-enriched milk. Add one tablespoon of low-fat powdered milk, a teaspoon of unpasteurized honey, a few drops of pure vanilla extract and a few fresh strawberries (wash and remove stems and caps). Instead of strawberries, you may use fresh peaches, peeled and sliced, or other fruit of your choice.

Blend the ingredients for a few seconds or until you have a smooth, frothy milk shake.

Osteoporosis

Osteoporosis, or porous bone, is a disease characterized by low bone mass and deterioration of bone. It leads to fragile bones and increased vulnerability to fractures, particularly of the spine, hip and wrist.

Because bone loss usually occurs without symptoms, osteoporosis is often called 'the silent disease'. People may not know that they have the condition until their bones become so weak that a sudden bump, a strain or a fall causes a vertebra to collapse or a bone to break.

Factors that increase the likelihood of osteoporosis developing include: having a thin and/or small frame; advanced age; post-menopause; having anorexia or bulimia nervosa; a diet low in calcium, vitamin D and other essential nutrients; lack of regular exercise, cigarette smoking and excessive use of alcohol.

Recommended measures for helping to prevent osteoporosis include:

- An adequate diet, rich in calcium, vitamin D and other essential nutrients, and low in refined, overprocessed foods.
- Chewing your food thoroughly, to facilitate proper digestion and assimilation of nutrients.
- A health-promoting lifestyle, with no smoking and with limited alcohol and caffeine intake.
- Avoiding the use of antacids that contain aluminium. They tend to leach calcium from the bones and cause the body to excrete it.
- Regular exercise, particularly weight-bearing exercise such as walking, running, dancing and playing tennis.

Copper

Copper helps in the proper functioning of nerve, brain and connective tissue. It is also essential for healthy blood and for the utilization of vitamin C.

If you regularly consume green leafy vegetables and whole grain products, you are unlikely to be copper deficient. Other good sources of this nutrient are: nuts, organ meats, prunes, pulses, seafood and seeds.

Fluoride

Fluoride has long been known to have an effect on bone. Epidemiological studies have shown increased bone density in people living in areas with a higher fluoride content in the drinking water, compared with those who live in areas where low-fluoride water is supplied. Fluoride works with calcium to strengthen bones.

Organic fluoride is found in almonds, beetroot tops, carrots, cheese, garlic, green vegetables, milk, steel-cut oats and sunflower seeds. It is also usually present in naturally hard water.

Manganese

The highest concentrations of manganese in the human body are in the bones and endocrine glands. Various studies provide evidence that this mineral plays an important role in bone health. Anyone interested in preventing osteoporosis should therefore make a conscious effort to consume adequate amounts of manganese.

Manganese is also essential for the utilization of vitamin C and the B vitamins, and for the synthesis of cartilage.

Foods rich in manganese include: beets, brown rice and the bran of brown rice (known as rice polish), egg yolk, green leafy vegetables, meats, nuts, peas, seaweed, seeds and wholegrain cereals.

Magnesium

As much as 50 per cent of all the magnesium in the body is found in the bones.

Magnesium is necessary for the metabolism of calcium, phosphorus, potassium, sodium and vitamin C, and for the synthesis of protein. It is also essential for effective nerve and muscle function.

Some multivitamin-mineral preparations contain magnesium and calcium in the right proportion, that is, half as much magnesium as calcium.

The best food sources of this mineral include: alfalfa sprouts, almonds, apples, dark green and other vegetables, figs, grapefruit, lemons, nuts, oranges, peas, potatoes, seeds, soya beans and yellow corn.

Phosphorus

Phosphorus is needed for sound bones and for a healthy nervous system. Many people obtain plenty of this mineral, which is abundant in foods such as meats and soft drinks. But nutritionists are concerned about diets that provide much more phosphorus than calcium, as this encourages bone loss. The key, therefore, is to consume more calcium-rich foods and less red meat. Commendable phosphorus sources include: corn, dried fruits, egg yolk, low-fat dairy products, nuts, pulses, seeds and whole grains.

Silica

Silica is an essential nutrient which must be constantly supplied from food sources. It plays an important part in many body functions and has a direct relationship to mineral absorption.

Bones are made up mainly of calcium, magnesium and phosphorus, but they also contain silica. Silica is essential for both the hardness and the flexibility of bones, and it is silica that is responsible for the depositing of minerals, especially calcium, into the bones. Moreover, silica hastens the healing of fractures and reduces scarring at fracture sites. Silica also contributes to the building up of connective tissue, and a deficiency leads to a weakening of the tissue.

Along with regular exercise, silica supplementation may be worth considering for the relief of aching and ageing joints, and to alleviate certain intestinal upsets which may be related to lower back pain. Two to four organic flavonoid chelated silica tablets or organic vegetal silica capsules daily with meals is the usual dosage, as a supplement to silica-rich foods. But first check with your doctor, naturopathic physician or other qualified health professional.

Spring horsetail (Equisetum arvense), better known as horsetail or scouring rush, is a perennial that grows wild in temperate zones. It is a rich natural source of organic silicates, from which vegetal silica is derived. Pure aqueous extract of vegetal silica from spring horsetail is 100 per cent water soluble and can therefore be completely absorbed by the body.

Caution: Ground horsetail is *not* suitable for this purpose as it can be abrasive to the intestinal tract.

Foods rich in silica include: barley, brown rice, corn, oats, millet, rye, sunflower seeds and whole wheat; fresh fruits and vegetables such as apples, cherries, pears, strawberries, asparagus, celery, green leafy vegetables, Jerusalem artichoke, kale, lettuce, onions, parsley, potatoes, red beets and red and green peppers.

Zinc

Zinc is a vital component of the immune system which protects us from disease. It is intricately involved in tissue nutrition and repair, and speeds up the healing of wounds.

Zinc is essential for the proper functioning of more than 70 enzyme systems and is also necessary for the assimilation of the B vitamins.

In addition, zinc plays a role in maintaining bone health. It enhances the biochemical actions of vitamin D, which is involved in calcium absorption and osteoporosis prevention.

There is evidence that zinc deficiency is relatively common in industrialized countries: the refining of sugar and flour results in substantial losses of this mineral. Elderly individuals are probably at increased risk of zinc deficiency because both their food intake and their ability to absorb nutrients tend to diminish with advancing age.

Foods rich in zinc include: brewer's yeast, cheese, eggs, broad (lima) beans, green beans, mushrooms, non-fat dry milk, nuts, poultry, pulses, pumpkin seeds, soya beans, sunflower seeds, wheat germ and wholegrain products.

Other Nutrients

Water

Not usually thought of as a nutrient, water is nevertheless the most important substance we consume. It is the principal constituent of body fluids. It is also the medium by which nutrients are transported to cells and wastes removed from the body. It is a lubricant and a shock absorber. It is essential for maintaining the moisture in the spinal discs, which cushion the vertebrae. It is necessary for proper digestion and for regulating body temperature. It is, in addition, useful in helping to prevent dehydration and constipation.

Our bones contain about 22 per cent water and the spinal discs about 80 per cent, and so an adequate daily water intake is crucial to spinal health. Eight to ten glasses of water is the ideal.

All liquids provide water, but some of the best sources are: unsweetened juices, non-caffeinated drinks such as herbal teas and milk and mineral water.

Protein

Protein forms the basic structure of all cells and a deficiency will result in loss of muscle mass and tone.

Protein is also essential for the synthesis of collagen, which is the basic material of bone. The body can create some protein building blocks (amino acids) but some must also come from protein in the diet.

High-protein diets, however, can cause you to lose more calcium in urine and faeces than you normally would. Osteoporosis, for example, is more common in parts of the world where dietary protein intake is high. An excess of protein also increases the need for other nutrients such as the B vitamins.

There are two types of protein. The first – complete protein – is obtained mainly from foods of animal origin such as eggs, dairy products, meat, poultry and seafood. They contain a proper balance of the eight essential amino acids. The other type – incomplete protein – lacks some essential amino acids but, in certain combinations, can be made complete. They are found in grains, pulses and seeds. Examples of combinations to render them complete are: rice and pulses; maize (corn) and beans; wholewheat bread with baked beans.

Carbohydrates

Natural complex carbohydrates, as provided by wholegrain breads and pasta, fresh fruits, fresh corn and other vegetables, are rich in nutrients. They are more slowly released from the stomach than the simple carbohydrates obtained from refined foods such as white flour, white rice and white sugar.

Complex carbohydrates furnish bulk, which appeases appetite and counteracts constipation which sometimes contributes to lower backache. Complex carbohydrates, moreover, promote a trim body and so discourage overweight and obesity, both of which are linked to back problems.

- For breakfast, try porridge or a high-fibre, low-sugar breakfast cereal. Add sliced banana or other fresh fruit if you wish, or sultanas or raisins. As part of your breakfast you may eat a couple of slices of wholegrain toast, but go lightly on the butter or margarine.
- For snacks, eat wholegrain bread rolls, crispbreads, muffins, fresh fruits, fresh vegetables or wholegrain breakfast cereal.
- For lunch, eat a nutritious sandwich made of wholegrain bread or have a baked potato with a low-fat topping (such as baked beans), pasta, brown rice or some other wholegrain food.
- For supper, make some brown rice, pasta and vegetables the main part of the meal.
- Fresh fruit is best for dessert.
- Take care not to add too much fat of any kind to your food. Complex carbohydrates have less than half the calories of fat. They are therefore unlikely to increase body weight, unless eaten excessively and with much fat added.

Fat

Fat is needed in the daily diet to provide energy, conserve body heat and help cells to function normally. Fat supports and protects vital organs and acts as a medium for the transport of fat-soluble vitamins (A, D, E and K).

Among the best sources of fat are: modest amounts of extra virgin olive oil, flaxseed oil, unrefined sesame and sunflower oils, organic butter and fish oils. These help the body to retain vitamin D and prevent calcium from being excreted in the urine. Other good sources of dietary fat include cheese, eggs, milk, nuts and seeds.

Nutrient antagonists

Nutrient antagonists are agents that act against the health-promoting properties of the vitamins, minerals and other nutrients provided by the food you eat.

Notable nutrient antagonists include:

- The regular taking of acetylsalicylic acid (Aspirin), which increases the need for vitamin C.
- Contraceptive pill, which can act against the B-complex vitamins and zinc.
- Rancid oils and other rancid food, which can destroy vitamin E in the body.
- Some commercial laxatives, if they are used regularly, as they can lead to deficiencies of vitamin C and the B vitamins.
- Regular use of antacids, which can impair the absorption of nutrients.
- Smoking, which destroys vitamin C and the B vitamins, and reduces vital oxygen supplies to the tissues.
- High alcohol intake, which is antagonistic to several of the essential vitamins and minerals that the body needs. It also contributes to weight gain as it supplies extra calories.
- Too much salt (sodium), which has been linked to high blood pressure.
- Too much caffeine, which promotes dehydration and robs the body of certain essential nutrients such as calcium.
- High-protein diets, which leach calcium and other nutrients from the body.

In a Nutshell: Diet for a Healthy Back

- Eat from a variety of nutrient-rich foods such as those mentioned in this chapter. Avoid overprocessed foods devoid of health-promoting nutrients.
- Avoid high-protein diets.
- Reduce your intake of high-fat and high-salt foods.
- Choose complex rather than simple carbohydrates.
- Cut down on caffeine and alcohol.
- Drink plenty of water.
- Be wary of nutrient antagonists (*see* page 42).
- Eat slowly to aid digestion and facilitate absorption of nutrients. Do not overeat.
- Shop wisely: build your meals around fresh fruits, fresh vegetables and wholegrain products. Store and cook your purchases so as to conserve nutrients.

Warming Up and Cooling Down | 4

Experts agree that regular, appropriate exercise is essential for the prevention of back problems and for preserving the health of the spine. Before doing exercises, however, adequate warming up is essential.

Warm-ups prepare the heart muscle for exercise. They stretch the skeletal muscles, which cover the body's bony framework, and help to reduce stiffness. They improve flexibility, they increase body temperature and improve blood and lymph circulation. They help to prevent muscular pulls and strain once the main exercises are in progress.

The warm-up exercises which follow have been selected because they are simple yet effective for limbering up the body. Several of them are also useful as tension relievers. They help to prevent a build-up of tension which could lead to aches and pains. These warm-ups can be readily incorporated into daily schedules. For example, the neck, shoulder and ankle exercises can be done during breaks from prolonged sitting at a computer, desk or machine, or at stops at rest areas during a long car journey. The *Rock-and-Roll* (*see* page 55) can be done on coming home from work, before tackling evening chores. Be on the lookout for opportunities to integrate these and similar exercises into your daily activities.

Before Starting

Before attempting to do the warm-up exercises or the exercises in chapter five, please check with your doctor or other health-care professional. Ask for an evaluation of your condition and for advice about the exercises in this book.

Once you have permission to do the exercises, you can be confident that they are suitable for you and compatible with any treatment you may be having. This is especially important if you have had surgery, if you have osteoporosis, arthritis or a spinal problem, or if you are pregnant.

If you have spondylolysis or spondylolisthesis, avoid forward-bending postures which can actually aggravate symptoms related to damaged vertebrae. (Spondylolysis is the breaking down of a vertebra and spondylolisthesis is the forward slipping of a vertebra.)

The same caution applies to people with osteoporosis, because the forces of flexion (bending forwards) place stress on the front of the vertebral bodies (block-shaped portion of the vertebrae, located at the front of the spine) and may cause fracture. Those who have had spinal fractures should also avoid these flexion exercises.

Please also study chapters one and two before trying to do the exercises. Modify the exercises, if necessary, to suit personal needs, and discontinue them at the first hint of discomfort or pain.

In addition, do consult with your health-care advisor if you experience any worsening of symptoms, such as pain, nausea, weakness or numbness after you begin to practise the exercises.

General Instructions

The following instructions pertain not only to the exercises in this chapter, but also to all the other exercises in this book.

Practise all the exercises with awareness and in synchronization with regular breathing. If they are done in this way, you are unlikely to strain or hurt yourself and you will also derive maximum benefit from them.

If you have to interrupt your regular practice, for example because of illness, restart gradually and be patient. Begin with the simplest warm-ups and postures and work towards the more challenging ones.

When to practise

Try to practise daily, but if this is not possible, practise every other day so as not to lose the benefits gained from your previous exercise session. It is also better to exercise for ten minutes every day than to do so for half an hour only once a week. Try to do your exercises at about the same time every day, or every other day, so as to establish and maintain a good habit.

Practising in the morning helps to reduce stiffness which can occur after many hours of lying in bed and also gives energy for the day's work. Practising in the evening produces a healthy fatigue and promotes good quality sleep. If you find evening exercise too stimulating, however, try to fit your exercises in where they prove most convenient and beneficial.

Several of the exercises, such as the neck, shoulder and ankle warm-ups, and many of the breathing exercises in chapter eight can be done at odd moments throughout the day to prevent tension from accumulating. You can tighten your abdominal muscles on an exhalation when standing in an elevator or sitting in a waiting-room. You can rotate your ankles when watching television, with your feet elevated. You can check your posture when you pass a mirror or shop window. You can do breathing exercises when driving or waiting in a queue or even at meetings or parties.

Food and drink

If you plan to exercise in the morning, when the blood sugar level is low, you may drink a glass of juice or eat something light, such as a slice of wholegrain bread, rather than exercise on a completely empty stomach.

Safety and comfort

Before starting to exercise, remove from your person any object that may cause pressure or injury, such as glasses or jewellery. Wear comfortable, loose-fitting clothing which allows you to breathe and move freely. If exercising during breaks at work, loosen your collar, belt and tie. Practise barefooted whenever possible, provided that it is safe to do so.

Empty your bladder and, if possible, your bowel before beginning the exercises. Take a warm (not hot) bath or shower – if this is convenient or desirable – to counteract any stiffness you may be experiencing. Rinse or clean your mouth and nasal passages.

Where to practise

For your exercises, choose a place where you will be free of interruptions for the duration of your practice. You may, for example, do neck and shoulder warm-ups in a parked car at your place of work if you can do so inconspicuously. Ensure that ventilation is good and lighting adequate but not harsh.

Practise on an even surface, carpeted or covered with a non-skid mat. Practise out of doors whenever you can, on a porch or lawn for example. I shall refer to this surface as the 'mat' in the exercise instructions.

The key words to guide you in your exercise practice are 'slowly' and 'consciously'. Keep your focus of attention on each movement as you perform it and synchronize it with regular breathing. This ensures delivery of oxygen to the working muscles and helps to eliminate substances that produce fatigue. **Do not** hold your breath. Rest briefly after you have completed each exercise, to prevent stiffness and a build-up of fatigue. At the end of your exercise session, be sure to cool down (see the relevant section at the end of this chapter).

When you first attempt to do the exercises do not be discouraged if your body does not immediately respond as you had hoped it would. Be patient and persevere. Do not force a position. With regular practice, you will see good results in a surprisingly short time.

Warm-up Exercises

The Neck

The following exercises, done slowly and with awareness, in synchronization with regular breathing, are wonderful for keeping the cervical (neck) part of the spine flexible and healthy.

Head Turns

1 Sit or stand comfortably, with the crown of your head uppermost. Relax your jaw, shoulders, arms and hands. Breathe regularly through your nose.
2 Slowly and smoothly turn your head to the right, as far as you can without strain (Fig. 20).
3 Slowly and smoothly turn your head to the left, as far as you can without strain (Fig. 21).
4 Turn your head to face forwards.
5 Repeat the exercise several times. Rest.

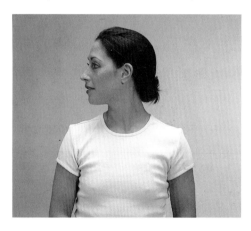

Fig. 20. Head Turn to the right

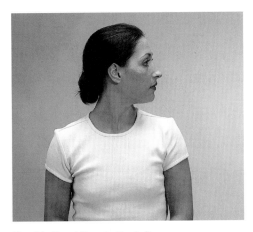

Fig. 21. Head Turn to the left

Ear-to-Shoulder

Sit comfortably. Close your eyes or leave them open. Keep your shoulders, arms and hands relaxed. Breathe regularly throughout the exercise. Tilt your head sideways as if to touch your shoulder with your ear (Fig. 22).

Bring your head upright. Tilt your head towards the opposite shoulder. Bring your head upright. Repeat the exercise a few times in smooth succession.

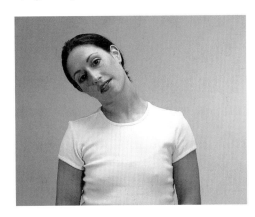

Fig. 22. Ear-to-Shoulder

The shoulders

The following shoulder exercises enhance the effects of the preceding neck exercises, as well as conditioning the upper back.

Shrugging

Sit comfortably erect. Keep your head still and your eyes open or closed. Breathe regularly throughout the exercise.

Pull your shoulders upwards (shrug) as if to touch your ears with them (Fig. 23). Hold the shrug briefly (*do not* hold your breath), then relax your shoulders. Repeat the exercise a few times.

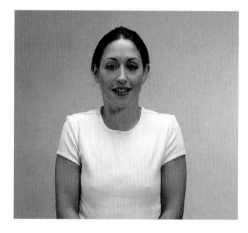

Fig. 23. Shrugging

Rotating

Sit comfortably erect. Keep your head still and your eyes open or closed. Breathe regularly throughout the exercise.

Pull your shoulders downwards and backwards, squeezing your shoulder blades together. Bring them forwards and upwards, then backwards and downwards to complete one rotation.

Repeat the rotation several times in smooth succession, then repeat the rotations a few times in reverse.

The Lying Twist

The is an exercise in torsion (twisting), which is beneficial to the abdominal muscles and to the lumbar part of the spine.

1   Lie on your back, with your arms sideways at shoulder level. Breathe regularly.
2   Bend your legs, one at a time, so that the soles of the feet are flat on the mat.
3   Bring the bent knees towards the chest.
4   Keeping the shoulders and arms in firm contact with the mat, *slowly, gently* and *smoothly* tilt the bent knees to one side as you exhale. You may keep your head still or you may turn it to the side opposite the tilted knees (Fig. 24).
5   Inhale and bring your knees back to the centre.
6   Exhale and tilt the knees to the other side, keeping the head still or turning it opposite to the tilted knees, as preferred. Be sure to keep your shoulders pressed to the mat.
7   Repeat the side-to-side tilting of the knees, several times in slow, smooth succession.
8   Stretch out and rest.

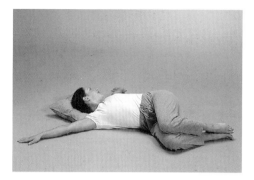

Fig. 24. Lying Twist

Having worked from the neck downwards, you are now ready to warm up the hip joints and legs. An excellent exercise for this is the *Butterfly*, and you will find it in chapter seven, Fig. 97 and 98, pages 112 and 113.

The ankles

Rotating

Sit where you can move your feet freely. Observe good posture. Breathe regularly. Rotate your ankles in slow, smooth circles (Fig. 25). Repeat the rotations in the opposite direction.

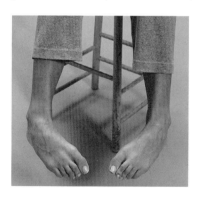

Fig. 25. Rotating ankles

Rock-and-Roll

This is an excellent all-over warm-up that not only conditions the back and abdominal muscles but also helps to loosen tight hamstrings. You may recall that the hamstring muscles, located at the back of the legs, contribute to the tilt of the pelvis and so are important contributors to good posture (*see* chapter one, page 7).

As an added benefit, when you practise the *Rock-and-Roll*, you press on 64 traditional acupuncture points.

This exercise should be done on a firm, even, well-padded surface.

1 Sit on your mat. Bend your legs and place the soles of your feet flat on the mat, close to your bottom.
2 Pass your arms *under* your bent knees and hug your thighs. Tuck your head down and chin in; make your back as rounded as you comfortably can. Breathe regularly.
3 On an inhalation, kick backwards to help you to roll onto your back (Fig. 26).
4 On an exhalation, kick forwards to come up again into a sitting position. Do *not* land heavily onto your feet as this will jar your spine. Simply touch the mat lightly with your toes.
5 Repeat the rock-and-roll movements several times in smooth succession, in synchronization with regular breathing.
6 Sit or lie down and rest.

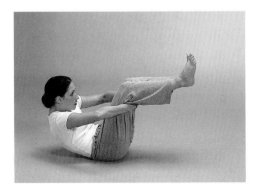

Fig. 26. Rock-and-Roll

Sun Salutations

This sequence of yoga postures is particularly beneficial for the maintenance of all-round spinal health. The twelve movements of the sequence exercise the spine forwards and backwards, and provide excellent leg stretches as well. They may be used not only as warm-ups, but also as cool-down exercises.

1 Stand tall, with the palms of your hands together, as if in prayer (Fig. 27). Breathe regularly.

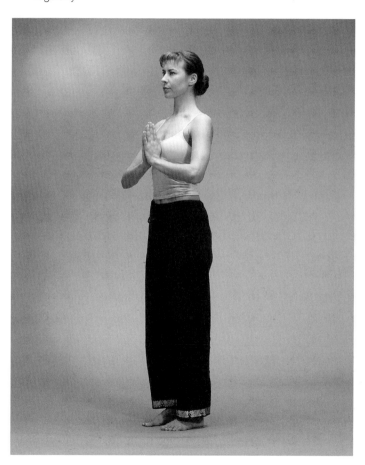

Fig. 27. Starting position

2 *Inhale* and carefully bend backwards to stretch the front of your body. Tighten your buttock muscles to help to protect your back (Fig. 28).

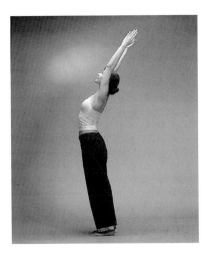

Fig. 28. Backward bend

3 *Exhale* and bend forwards – at the hip joints rather than at the waist – and place your hands on the mat beside your feet (Fig. 29). If necessary bend your knees; as you become more flexible you will be able to execute this step with knees straight.

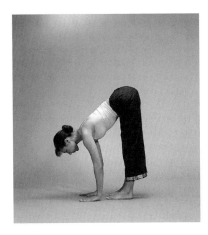

Fig. 29. Forward bend

4   *Inhale* and look up. Taking the weight of your body on both hands, step back with your right foot (toes point forwards) (Fig. 30).

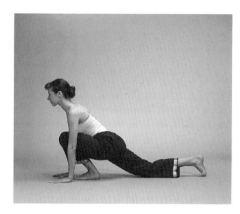

Fig. 30. Leg stretch

5   Briefly suspending your breath (neither inhaling nor exhaling), also step backwards with your left foot. The weight of your body is now borne by your hands and feet, and your body is level from the back of your head to your heels (Fig. 31).

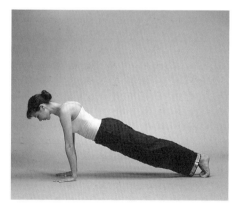

Fig. 31. Level body position

6   *Exhale* and lower your knees to the mat. Also lower your chin (or forehead – whichever is more comfortable) and chest to the mat (Fig. 32).

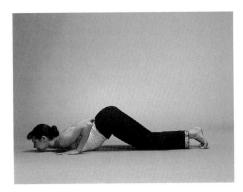

Fig. 32. Knee-chest position

7   *Inhaling*, relax your feet so that your toes point backwards. Lower your body to the mat and *slowly and carefully* arch your back. Keep your head up and back, and your hands pressed to the mat (Fig. 33). This is the *Cobra* position, which is again described in chapter five, page 82 in more detail, as a separate exercise.

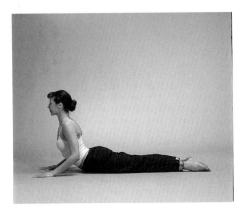

Fig. 33. Cobra

8   *Exhale* and point your toes forwards; push against the mat with your hands to help to raise your hips. Keep your arms straight (or almost straight) and hang your head down. Aim your heels towards the mat but do not strain your leg muscles (Fig. 34). This is the *Dog Stretch* posture, which is again described in chapter seven, page 118, as a separate exercise.

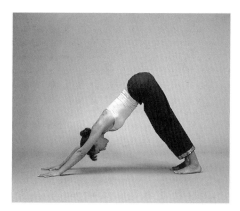

Fig. 34. Dog stretch

9   *Inhaling*, look up, rock forwards onto your toes and step between your hands with your left foot (Fig. 35).

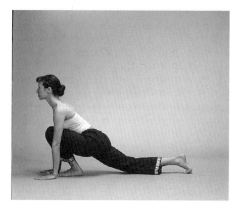

Fig. 35. Leg stretch

10 *Exhaling*, step between your hands with your right foot and bend forwards (Fig. 36).

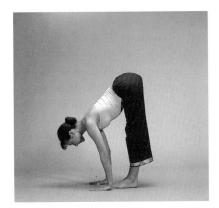

Fig. 36. Forward bend

12 *Inhaling*, come up carefully into a standing position and move smoothly into a backward bend (Fig. 37).

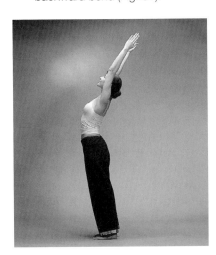

Fig. 37. Backward bend

13 *Exhale* and resume your starting position (Fig. 38). Breathe regularly.

Repeat all twelve movements as many times as you wish alternating your leading leg each time. Rest afterwards.

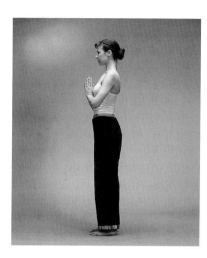

Fig. 38. Start/finish position

Cooling down

Cooling down after exercise affords a chance for static muscle stretching which enhances flexibility. It provides an activity for the cardiovascular system (heart and blood vessels) to return gradually to normal functioning after a period of exercise. It helps to prevent problems such as a drop in blood pressure, feelings of lightheadedness, dizziness and fainting, which can occur if you stop exercising abruptly.

Most of the exercises given in the section on warm-ups can also be done as cool-down exercises. You may also wish to try the following:

The Stick Posture

This is essentially an all-over body stretch done in a supine, or lying on the back, position.

1   Lie on your mat, with your legs stretched out in front and your arms at your sides. Close your eyes and breathe regularly.

2   Inhale slowly, smoothly and deeply as you bring your arms overhead and if possible, place your palms together. At the same time, stretch your legs to their fullest extent, pulling your toes towards you and pushing your heels away from you (Fig. 39). The entire stretch should be done as one smooth, conscious movement in synchronization with a slow inhalation.

3   Maintain the all-body stretch for a few seconds but *do not hold your breath*.

4   Exhale and release the all-over stretch, bringing your arms back at your sides. Rest.

5   You may repeat the exercise once. Rest afterwards.

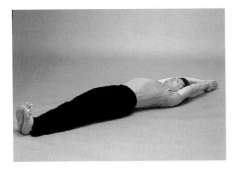

Fig. 39. Stick Posture – Lying

Standing version of the Stick Posture

1 Stand tall, with your weight equally distributed between your feet. Relax your arms at your sides. Breathe regularly.

2 Inhale and raise your arms overhead, stretching them fully. Bring your palms together if you can (Fig. 40).

3 Hold the all-body stretch for several seconds, but do not hold your breath.

4 Exhale and lower your arms to resume your starting position. Rest.

5 You may repeat the exercise once. Rest afterwards.

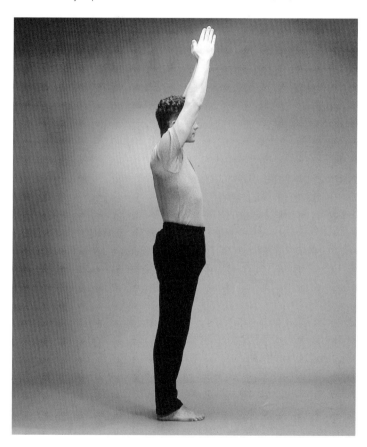

Fig. 40. Stick Posture – Standing

Toe-to-top relaxation (Savasana)

This exercise is a favourite of yoga students. It often marks the end of a yoga exercise session, and it is now frequently practised to promote deep relaxation.

The basic position is described in step 1, but you may modify this to suit your particular condition, preference or circumstances.

1 Lie on your back with your legs stretched out in front of you. Separate your feet to discourage a build-up of tension in your legs. Move your arms a little away from your sides to prevent an accumulation of tension in your shoulders. Keep your arms straight but relaxed, and your palms of your hands upturned. Close your eyes. Unclench your teeth to relax your jaw, but keep your mouth closed without compressing your lips. Breathe regularly (Fig. 41).

2 Focus your attention on your feet. Pull your toes towards you, pushing your heels away. Hold the ankle position briefly. Do *not* hold your breath. Keep breathing regularly throughout the exercise. Now relax your feet and ankles.

3 Stiffen your legs, locking your knee joints. Hold briefly. Relax your knees.

4 Tighten your buttock muscles. Hold the tightness for a few seconds. Release the tightness.

5 On an *exhalation*, press the small of your back (waist level) towards or against the mat. Hold the pressure as long as your exhalation lasts, then release the pressure as you inhale. Keep breathing regularly.

6 Inhale and squeeze your shoulderblades together. Hold the squeeze as long as the inhalation lasts. Release the squeeze as you exhale. Keep breathing regularly.

7 On an *exhalation*, tighten your abdominal muscles. Hold the tightness as long as the exhalation lasts. Inhale and relax. Keep breathing regularly.

8 Take a slow, smooth, deep inhalation, *without strain*, imagining that you are filling the top, middle and bottom of your lungs. Be aware of your chest expanding and your abdomen rising. Exhale slowly, smoothly and steadily, imagining that you are emptying your lungs by degrees. Be aware of your chest and abdomen relaxing. Resume regular breathing.

9 Tighten your hands into fists; straighten your arms; raise them off the mat. Hold the stiffness briefly, then let the arms and hands fall to the mat, free of stiffness. Relax them.

10 Keep your arms relaxed, but shrug your shoulders as if to touch your ears with them. Hold the shrug briefly, then relax your shoulders.

11 Gently roll your head from side to side a few times. Reposition your head. Keep breathing regularly.

12 Exhaling, open your eyes and mouth widely; stick your tongue out; tense all your facial muscles. Inhale, close your mouth and eyes and relax your facial muscles. Imagine your facial features becoming softer and more serene. Breathe regularly.

13 Lie relaxed for as many minutes as you can spare. Give your body weight up to the surface that supports it. Each time you exhale, let your body sink more deeply into that surface, increasingly relaxed.

14 Before getting up, rotate your ankles, roll your head gently from side to side and leisurely stretch your limbs. Do the *Lying Twist* (*see* Fig. 24, page 54) or whatever movements you feel like doing. Never get up suddenly. Rather, do so slowly and carefully, as suggested in chapter two, page 23, in the section entitled *Getting Up (from lying)*. Prepare to resume your usual activities with renewed energy.

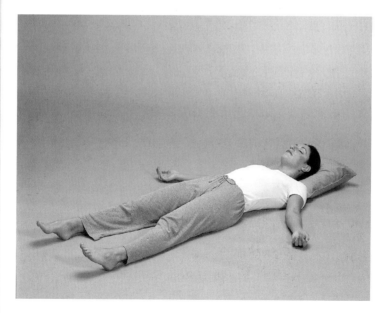

Fig. 41. Toe-to-top relaxation (Savasana)

Essential Back Exercises | 5

In chapter one, you read about the anatomy of the spine and about other structures connected with it. All these components work together, in health, to keep you upright yet give you the flexibility to move about efficiently. They enable you to bend forwards, backwards and sideways, and to twist, or rotate, your body. They also allow you to turn your head from side to side and to tilt it forwards and backwards.

The exercises that follow have been carefully selected to help to strengthen the back and structures relating to it; to promote spinal flexibility; to keep joints freely moving and to relax back muscles. A rigid back is more vulnerable to pain, stress and injury than a flexible one. Faithful practice of these exercises is therefore encouraged.

Before Starting

Before you begin to practise the back exercises in this chapter, please read the section entitled 'Before Starting' and all the sections under the heading 'General Instructions' in chapter four (pages 46 to 49).

Back Exercises

The Cat Stretch series

1 Get on your hands and knees in an 'all-fours' position (Fig. 42).

2 *Inhaling*, bend your elbows and lower your chest to the mat, taking care not to let your back sag. Keep your head back so that your neck receives a gentle, therapeutic stretch as your chin touches the mat. Let your arms and hands take most of the weight so as not to subject your back to unnecessary pressure. This is the 'knee-chest' position (Fig. 43).

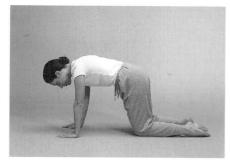

Fig. 42. Cat Stretch – 'all-fours' position

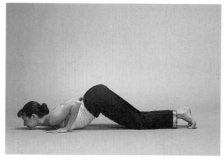

Fig. 43. Cat Stretch – 'knee-chest' position

3 On an *exhalation*, return to the all-fours position (Fig. 42). Breathe regularly.

4 On an *exhalation*, lower your head, make your back rounded and bring one knee toward your forehead. This is the 'knee-to-forehead' position (Fig. 44).

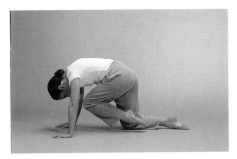

Fig. 44. Cat Stretch – 'knee-to-forehead' position

5   *Inhaling*, push the bent leg backwards, stretching it out fully and lifting it as high as absolutely comfortable; raise your head. This is the 'all-body stretch' (Fig. 45), which can be done without accentuating the inward curve of the back unnecessarily. Breathe regularly.

6   Exhale and lower your knee to the mat. Breathe regularly.

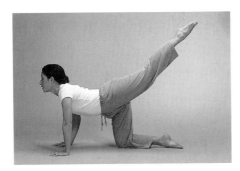

Fig. 45. Cat Stretch – 'all-body stretch'

7   Repeat the all-body stretch (Fig. 45), with the other leg. Exhale and lower your leg to the mat. Breathe regularly.

8   Lie on your back and rest, or relax in the *Pose of a Child* (Figs. 71 and 72, page 85).

Note well

If you have recently given birth, *please check with your doctor* before practising the knee-chest position of the Cat Stretch series (Fig. 43). If you practise this exercise earlier than six weeks post-natally, you risk introducing bubbles (air emboli) into your circulatory system.

The Pelvic Tilt Lying

1   Lie on your back with your legs outstretched in front.
2   Slide your hands under your waist. You will note a hollow – the lumbar arch of your spine (Fig. 46).

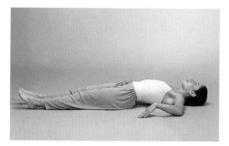

Fig. 46. Preparing for Pelvic Tilt Lying – showing lumbar arch

3   Now relax your arms and hands at your sides. Bend your legs and rest the soles of your feet flat on the mat, at a comfortable distance from your bottom. Breathe regularly. On an *exhalation*, press the small of your back (waist) towards or against the mat to eliminate the hollow you felt there (Fig. 47). As you do so, you will note that your pelvis tilts gently upwards.
4   Hold the downwards pressure of the waist as long as your exhalation lasts.
5   Inhale and relax.
6   You may repeat the exercises once now, and again later. Stretch out and rest afterwards.

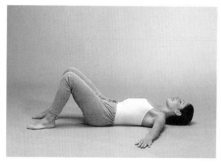

Fig. 47. Pelvic Tilt Lying – without lumbar arch

1. Get on all-fours (Fig. 48). Exhale and tuck your bottom down. Lower your head. Make your back as rounded as possible (Fig. 49).
2. Hold the posture briefly, but *do not* hold your breath.
3. Inhale and resume your starting position. Breathe regularly.
4. You may repeat the exercise once now, and again later.

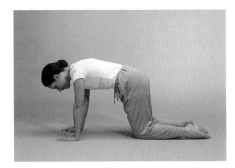

Fig. 48. Pelvic Tilt on All-fours – back level

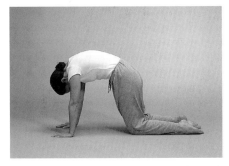

Fig. 49. Pelvic Tilt on All-fours – hips down

Variation: The Pelvic Tilt Sitting

1 Sit naturally erect on a chair with a straight back. Rest the soles of your feet flat on the floor (Fig. 50).

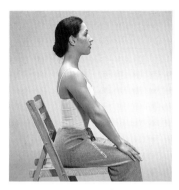

Fig. 50. Pelvic Tilt Sitting – showing lumbar arch

2 On an *exhalation*, press the back of your waist firmly towards or against the back of the chair (Fig. 51).

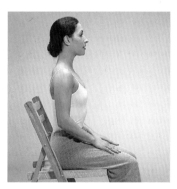

Fig. 51. Pelvic Tilt Sitting – no lumbar arch

3 Hold the pressure as long as exhalation lasts.
4 Inhale and relax. Breathe regularly.
5 You may repeat the exercise once now, and again later.

1   Stand naturally erect, with your back against a wall or other suitable prop (Fig. 52).

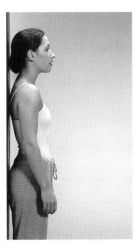

Fig. 52. Pelvic Tilt Standing – lumbar arch

2   *Exhale* and press the back of your waist towards or against the prop (Fig. 53).
3   Hold the pressure as long as exhalation lasts.

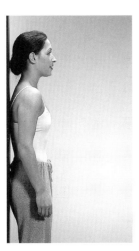

Fig. 53. Pelvic Tilt Standing – without lumbar arch

4   Inhale and relax.

5   You may repeat the exercise once now, and again later.

Notes

Opportunities for practising an appropriate version of the Pelvic Tilt are countless. Examples are: during television commercial breaks; while waiting for the kettle to boil; during breaks on a long car or bus journey; during tea or coffee breaks at your place of work (in the lounge, washroom or behind closed doors elsewhere in the building); against the wall of a lift (elevator) – no one will know what you're doing.

The Bridge

1. Lie on your back with your legs bent and the soles of your feet flat on the mat, comfortably close to your bottom. Relax your arms close to your sides, with your palms turned downwards. Breathe regularly.

2. *Inhaling*, raise first your hips, then slowly and smoothly the middle of your back until your torso is off the mat (Fig. 54). *Do not* arch the small of your back. Your feet, arms and hands, upper back and head remain in firm contact with the mat.

3. Hold the raised-torso posture as long as it is comfortable for you. Keep breathing regularly.

4. Slowly and smoothly lower your torso, *in reverse* motion, as if curling your spine one bone at a time, onto the mat. Synchronize your breathing with this movement.

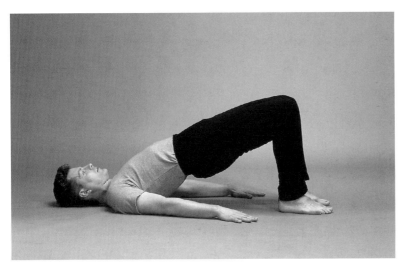

Fig. 54. The Bridge

Variation: The Bridge

1 Lie on your back with your legs bent and the soles of your feet flat on the mat, comfortably close to your bottom. Relax your arms close to your sides, with your palms turned downwards. Breathe regularly.

2 *Inhaling*, raise first your hips, then slowly and smoothly the middle of your back until your torso is off the mat. Do not arch the small of your back. Your feet, arms, hands, upper back and head remain in firm contact with the mat.

3 Stretch your arms overhead to their comfortable limit (Fig. 55).

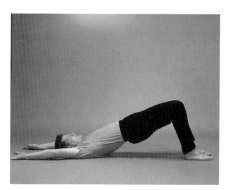

Fig. 55. The Bridge – arms extended

4 Hold the posture for as long as you comfortably can. Keep breathing regularly.

5 Bring your arms back to the side of your body and turn your palms downwards. Slowly and smoothly lower your torso in reverse motion, as if curling your spine, one bone at a time, onto the mat. Synchronize this movement with regular breathing. Rest.

Knee Press

1 Lie on your back with your legs stretched out in front and your arms and hands relaxed beside you. Breathe regularly.
2 *Exhaling*, bend one leg and bring the bent knee towards you. Clasp your hands around the bent knee (Fig. 56). This is the basic knee press.
3 Hold the posture as long as you wish, breathing regularly.
4 Return to the starting position.
5 Repeat the exercise with the other leg.
6 Repeat the entire exercise, if you wish.

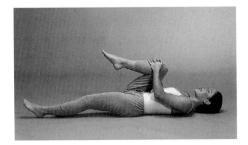

Fig. 56. Basic Knee Press

Knee Press (variation I)

1 Lie on your back with your legs stretched out in front and your arms and hands relaxed beside you. Breathe regularly.
2 *Exhaling*, bend one leg and bring the knee towards you. Clasp your hands around the bent knee. *Carefully* raise your head and bring the forehead towards the bent knee (Fig. 57).
3 Hold the posture as long as you wish, breathing regularly.
4 Carefully lower your head to the mat. Lower your leg to the mat and resume your starting position.
5 Repeat the exercise with the other leg.
6 Repeat the entire exercise, if you wish.

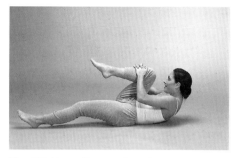

Fig. 57. Knee Press – head raised

Knee Press (variation II)

1   Lie on your back with your legs stretched out in front and your arms and hands relaxed beside you. Breathe regularly.
2   *Exhaling*, bend one leg and bring the knee towards you. Continue breathing regularly.
3   Again on an *exhalation*, bend your other leg and bring it towards you. Continue breathing regularly. Hold the bent legs securely.
4   Carefully raise your head and bring your forehead towards the bent knees as you exhale. Keep your shoulders as relaxed as possible (Fig. 58).
5   Hold the posture as long as you comfortably can, breathing regularly.
6   *Carefully* lower your head to the mat.
7   Release the hold on each leg in turn and carefully lower it to the mat.
8   Rest, breathing regularly.

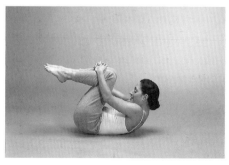

Fig. 58. Knee Press – both knees and head raised

The Star Posture

1 Sit comfortably erect with your legs stretched out in front. Breathe regularly.
2 Bend one leg and place the sole of the foot flat on the mat opposite the knee of the outstretched leg (Figs. 59 and 60). This establishes the distance between the feet and rest of the body once you are performing the exercise.

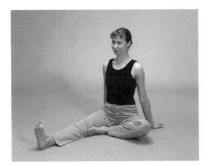

Fig. 59. The Star Posture – right leg straight, front view

3 Bend your outstretched leg. Place the two soles together (Fig. 61).
4 Clasp your hands securely around your feet.

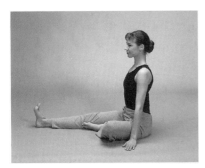

Fig. 60. The Star Posture – right leg straight, side view

5 *Exhaling*, bend forwards slowly, smoothly and with control, bringing your face towards your feet. Once you have reached your comfortable limit, relax your head downwards (Fig. 62).

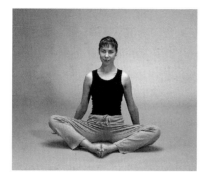

Fig. 61. The Star Posture – both knees bent

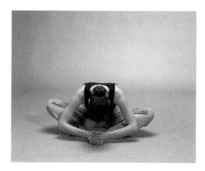

Fig. 62. The Star Posture – completed posture with head down

6   Hold the posture for as long as you are comfortable in it while breathing regularly.

7   Slowly resume your starting position, synchronizing movement with breathing.

8   Lie down and rest.

The Cobra

This posture was described as part of the *Sun Salutations* (see chapter four, Fig. 33, page 59), but it will be repeated here in more detail, as a separate exercise.

1   Lie on your abdomen, with your head turned to the side. Relax your arms and hands beside you (Fig. 63). Breathe regularly.

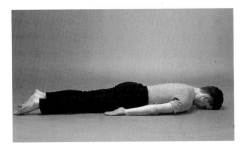

Fig. 63. The Cobra – lying down

2   Turn your head to the front, resting your forehead on the mat. Place the palms of your hands on the mat directly beneath your shoulders. Keep your arms close to your sides.
3   On an *inhalation*, bend your neck backwards, *slowly and carefully*: touch the mat with your nose then your chin in one smooth movement. Breathe regularly. Continue arching your spine: First the upper back (Fig. 64), then the lower back, in one fluid, graceful movement, until you can arch your back no farther. Keep your hips in contact with the mat throughout the exercise (Fig. 65).

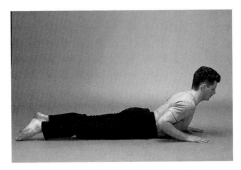

Fig. 64. The Cobra – midway arched back

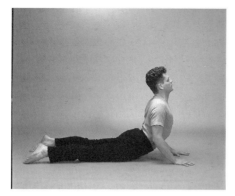

Fig. 65. The Cobra – completed posture, back arched, chin up

4   Maintain this posture for a few seconds, or as long as you can with absolute comfort. Keep breathing regularly.

5   Come out of the posture *in reverse, very slowly, smoothly and with control*: lower your abdomen to the mat, then lower your chest, chin, nose and forehead, in synchronization with regular breathing.

6   Relax your arms and hands beside you. Turn your head to the side (Fig. 66). Rest.

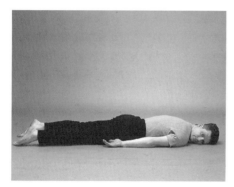

Fig. 66. The Cobra – recovery, lying with head to side
Following the *Cobra*, get onto all-fours and move into the *Pose of a Child*, which follows (Figs. 71 and 72).

1   Lie on your abdomen, with your legs slightly apart, and your arms relaxed at your side (Fig. 67). Breathe regularly.

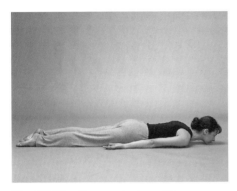

Fig. 67. The Bow – start position

2   Turn your head to the front and rest your forehead on the mat. Bend your knees and bring your feet towards your bottom (Fig. 68).

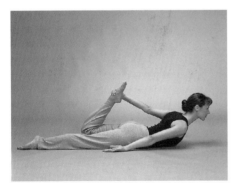

Fig 68. The Bow – head to front, knees bent

3   Carefully tilt your head backwards. Reach for your feet and grasp your ankles (Fig. 69).

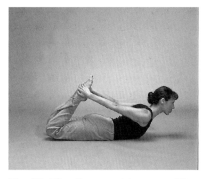

Fig. 69. The Bow – midway position

4   Exhale as you push your feet away and upwards. This action will raise your legs and arch your back (Fig. 70).

5   Maintain the posture only as long as you are absolutely comfortable in it. Keep breathing regularly.

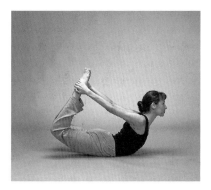

Fig. 70. The Bow – completed posture

6   Slowly and carefully ease yourself back onto the mat and resume your starting position. Rest while breathing regularly.

After completing *the Bow*, you may push yourself onto your hands and knees and move into the *Pose of a Child* (Figs. 71 and 72, page 85).

Pose of a Child

1 Sit in the *Japanese Sitting Position* (see chapter two, Fig. 9, page 13). Breathe regularly.
2 Slowly and carefully bend forwards, resting your forehead on the mat, or turning your face to the side. Relax your arms and hands beside you (Figs. 71 and 72).

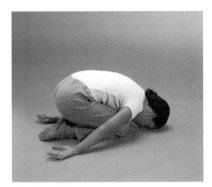

Fig. 71. Pose of a Child – side view

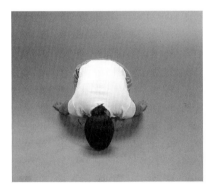

Fig. 72. Pose of a Child – front view

3 Stay in this posture for as long as you are comfortable in it. Continue breathing regularly.
4 Resume your starting position.

Pose of a Child – variation

Instead of resting your arms beside you, stretch them out ahead of you (Figs. 73 and 74).

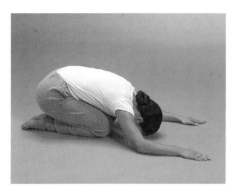

Fig. 73. Pose of a Child – variation, arms extended, side view

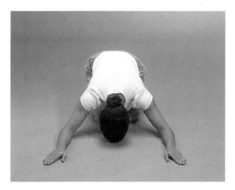

Fig. 74. Pose of a Child – variation, side view

Notes

- This is a good posture in which to rest after backward-bending poses such as the *Bridge* (Fig. 54, page 75), the *Cobra* (Fig. 63, page 81) and the *Bow* (Fig. 69, page 83).
- If you find it difficult for your head to reach the mat, place a cushion or pillow in front of you, on which to rest your forehead or face.

The Half-Moon

1 Stand naturally erect, with your feet close together, and your body weight equally distributed between them. Breathe regularly.
2 *Inhaling*, bring your arms upwards, pressing your palms together, if you can (Fig. 75). Keep your arms aligned with your ears.

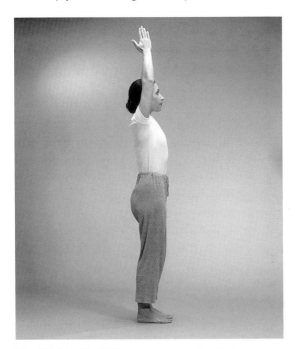

Fig. 75. The Half-Moon – arms extended

3 *Exhaling*, slowly and carefully bend to one side to form a graceful sideways arch of the body (Fig. 76).
4 Hold the posture for several seconds or as long as you comfortably can while breathing regularly.

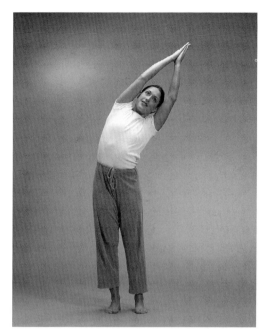

Fig. 76. The Half-Moon – completed posture

5　Inhale and return to the upright position. Exhale and lower your arms to your sides. Breathe regularly.

6　Repeat the exercise, bending to the other side.

7　Relax.

You may repeat the exercise if you wish.

The Spinal Twist

1   Sit naturally erect on your mat, with your legs stretched out in front of you (Fig. 77). Breathe regularly.

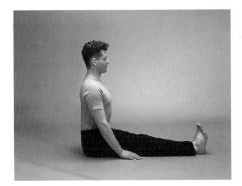

Fig. 77. Spinal Twist – legs straight in front

2   Bend your *left* leg at the knee and place your *left* foot beside the outer aspect of your *right* knee. Keep breathing regularly.
3   On an *exhalation*, *slowly and smoothly* twist your upper body to the *left* and rest both hands on the mat on your *left* side. Turn your head and look over your *left* shoulder (Fig. 78).

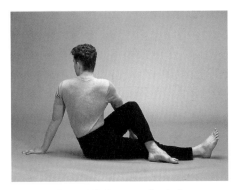

Fig. 78. Spinal Twist – to the left

4 Hold the posture for as long as you comfortably can. Keep breathing regularly.

5 Slowly untwist and return to your starting position. Rest briefly.

6 Repeat the twist to the right side, as follows: Stretch your left leg in front of you. Bend your right leg. Place your right foot beside the outer aspect of your left knee. As you exhale, slowly and carefully twist your upper body to the right and place both hands on the mat at your right side. Turn your head and look over your right shoulder (Fig. 79).

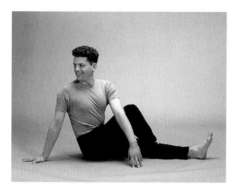

Fig. 79. Spinal Twist – to the right

7 Slowly untwist, stretch out your legs and rest.

Variation

When you become more flexible, you may wish to try this advanced version of the *Spinal Twist*.

1   Sit naturally erect on your mat, with your *right* leg stretched out in front and your *left* leg *folded inwards*.
2   Step over your folded leg with your *right* foot. *Exhale* and twist your upper body to the *right*. Rest both hands on the mat. Turn your head and look over your *right* shoulder (Fig. 80).
3   Maintain the posture for as long as you comfortably can. Keep breathing regularly.

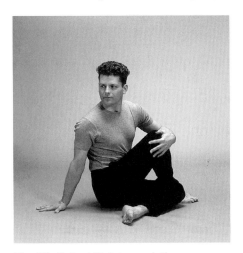

Fig. 80. Spinal Twist – variation

4   Slowly untwist and return to your starting position. Rest briefly.
5   Repeat the twist to the *left* side. Rest afterwards.

Pregnant women will welcome a gentler, more convenient spinal twist. You will find this described and illustrated in my book *Easy Pregnancy with Yoga* (*see* bibliography, page 188).

To complete these essential back exercises, please also practise the *Half Locust* (*see* chapter seven, Fig. 109, page 120).

Exercises to Strengthen your Abdomen and Support your Back

Not everyone knows that the abdominal muscles provide reinforcement to the muscles supporting the pelvis and spine. Many of you may be surprised to learn that the condition of muscles located at the front of your body may be related to discomfort or pain felt in the back. In fact, weak abdominal muscles are a common cause of backache.

The Abdominal Corset

As mentioned in chapter one, page 1, in order to drive a motor vehicle or operate a piece of machinery intelligently you need some familiarity with its workings; in the same way, you can't appreciate the role of the abdominal muscles and the principles underlying abdominal exercises without at least a basic knowledge of the structure and function of these muscles.

Here, then, is a pain-free lesson in the positions, attachments and functions of the principal abdominal muscles, sometimes incorrectly referred to, even by health professionals, as the 'stomach muscles'.

The *rectus abdominis* is a long, flat muscle that runs down the front of the abdomen, from the breastbone (sternum) to the pubic bones, on each side of an imaginary line drawn down the middle. It flexes the spine (as when bowing or bending forwards), and it supports the viscera (organs inside the abdomen).

The *obliquus externus abdominis* is a muscle with fibres running obliquely from the lower ribs to the iliac crest, which some people can feel as the front of the 'hip bone'. It flexes the trunk laterally (sideways), rotates it (as when twisting) and it also supports the viscera.

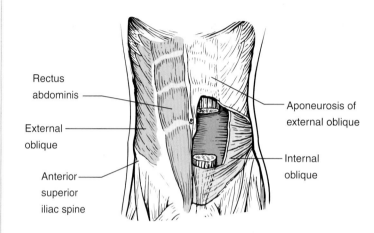

Rectus abdominis

External oblique

Anterior superior iliac spine

Aponeurosis of external oblique

Internal oblique

Fig. 81. The abdominal corset

The *obliquus internus abdominis* muscle is situated in the same place as the obliquus externus, but its fibres run in the opposite direction. These two sets of muscles are collaborators, working in harmony as one to produce the same actions.

The *transversalis abdominis* lies beneath the two preceding muscles, and its fibres run transversely as its name suggests. It assists the oblique abdominal muscles, just mentioned.

Finally, there are the *quadratus lumborum* muscles, lying on each side of the vertebral column (spine), and running from the last ribs to the iliac crest in front. They help the other abdominal muscles to perform their functions effectively.

The foregoing muscles are arranged like a four-way corset, spanning the front of the trunk from the breastbone and ribs to the public bones, and around the side of the ridge of the pelvis, which some people feel at each hip.

Although each muscle or set of muscles makes a contribution to the function of this abdominal corset, different sets work in combination during certain activities and exercises. For instance, the top half of the corset comes into play more noticeably than the bottom part during movements involving the upper trunk. When the legs are raised, however, it is the lower abdominals that are emphasized; they help to stabilize the pelvis.

Functions of the Abdominal Muscles

Here, for easy reference, is a summary of the functions of the muscles forming the four-way abdominal corset:

- To give support to the viscera (abdominal and pelvic organs).
- In collaboration with the buttock muscles (which pull downwards as the abdominals pull upwards), to control the tilt of the pelvis to maintain its correct alignment in relation to the spine.
- To flex the trunk sideways (half of the muscles are used).
- To raise the trunk upwards from a supine (lying on the back) or semi-supine position; even raising the head will cause the abdominal muscles to tighten.
- To rotate the trunk, as in bringing one shoulder towards the hip on the opposite side.
- To help to brace the body when it is being strained, as occurs during lifting or attempting to ward off blows. This is a reflex protective action.
- To help to stabilize the pelvis during leg raising.
- To assist in conscious acts of breathing; in coughing, sneezing, shouting and singing, and in elimination of body wastes; also during childbirth.

It is worth noting that sitting and standing postures provide little stimulus for abdominal muscles; nor does walking normally on level terrain. This is partly why the abdominals are usually the weakest group of muscles in people in industrialized societies. It is also partly the cause of the prevalence of backache. The abdominal muscles are afforded maximum exertion when they are required to perform against resistance, such as leverage and body weight. Other actions that effectively exercise the abdominals include trunk- and leg-raising from a horizontal position, running and lifting objects.

Essential principles for exercising abdominals

Before attempting practice of any abdominal exercises, it is a good idea to have some understanding of the principles underlying their action. Once you comprehend these principles, you will perform the exercises to follow more intelligently and therefore more safely; you will incur less risk of straining joints and muscles than if you practised in random fashion. You will also better appreciate chapter two, which deals with posture and body mechanics.

Most of the exercises in this chapter emphasize control of the tilt of the pelvis. This is because proper pelvic tilt improves posture and helps to prevent back strain.

The more advanced exercises challenge abdominal muscles to work against the resistance of gravity, thereby improving the condition and strength of the muscular abdominal corset, and eventually leading to the acquisition of optimum abdominal power.

Note well

Exercises such as raising and lowering the trunk and the legs do involve leverage and force of gravity for resistance. The consensus of experts, however, is that these exercises are often ineffective for strengthening the abdomen and are, in fact, potentially dangerous to the back. The actions involved in conventional sit-ups and double leg raising with legs straight depend largely on the flexor muscles of the hips, and frequently generate backache and back pain because they exert undue pull on joints of the lumbar spine.

Before starting

Please *check with your doctor* before doing these or any other exercises.

Please warm up before practising the exercises (*see* chapter four).

A note to pregnant woman

Except for the Abdominal Lift (Fig. 95), the exercises in this chapter are safe for most pregnant women to practise, as long as the doctor approves, and provided they feel comfortable to do. However, I suggest a look at my book entitled *Easy Pregnancy with Yoga* (*see* bibliography), which was written especially for the pre- and post-natal women.

Hints on sit-up exercises

- Almost all the abdomen-strengthening effect of a sit-up occurs from the first 30 to 45 degrees; after that, the hip flexors take over. Simply curling up 17.5 to 20 centimetres (7 to 8 inches), keeping your waist on the surface on which you are exercising, is enough to exercise the abdominal muscles.
- The knees should be bent and the soles of the feet supported (for example, by the floor). This flattens and protects the lower back.
- The feet should *not* be held down. If they are, it could conceal weakness of the abdominals, while the hip flexors do the work.
- It is important to do diagonal movements (such as the *Diagonal Curl-up*, Fig. 86, page 101), as well as straight up-and-down movements, to ensure exercise of all components of the muscular abdominal corset.
- Keep your chin tucked down; keep your back rounded rather than straight, since the latter promotes action of the hip flexors.
- Avoid jerking movements; curl up and down smoothly, in synchronization with regular breathing.

Preparing to exercise

Before practising the exercises to follow, be sure to warm up properly (*see* chapter four). Please also review the general instructions (also in chapter four) which apply to the practice of all the exercises described in chapters five, six and seven. Here, for quick reference, is a summary of these instructions.

- Wear loose, comfortable clothing that permits you to breathe and stretch easily.
- Practise the exercises on a firm, padded surface, such as a carpeted floor (referred to as the 'mat').
- Concentration is essential: practise the exercises slowly and with complete awareness. Synchronize movement with regular breathing.
- Once you have completed the exercise, with no strain whatever, maintain the posture for as many seconds as you wish, or can with absolute comfort (referred to as 'hold' the position).
- When holding the position, *do not* hold your breath; keep breathing naturally.
- When you are ready to come out of the posture, do so slowly and with awareness; synchronize movement with regular breathing.
- After completing the exercise, rest briefly before practising another exercise.

At the end of your exercise session, cool down adequately (see chapter four, pages 63 to 66 for suggestions).

The Exercises

The Yoga Sit-up

1 Lie on your back, with your legs stretched out and slightly separated (Fig. 82). Breathe regularly.

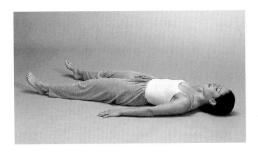

Fig. 82. Yoga Sit-up – lying down

2 Bend your knees and slide your feet towards your bottom until the soles are flat on the mat. (Maintain this distance between feet and bottom as you practise the sit-up.) Rest your palms on your thighs (Fig. 83).

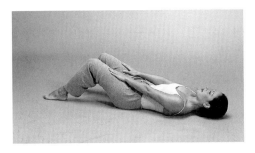

Fig. 83. Yoga Sit-up – palms on thighs

3 *Exhale* as you slowly and carefully raise your head. Keep your gaze on your hands as you slide them along your thighs, as if to touch your knees (Fig. 84).

4   When you feel maximum tolerable tension in your abdomen, stop and hold the posture for as long as you are absolutely comfortable in it. Keep breathing regularly.

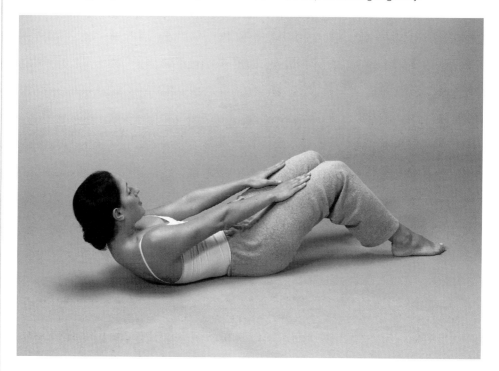

Fig. 84. Yoga Sit-up – completed posture

5   Inhale and resume your starting position by slowly curling your spine back onto the mat. Relax your arms and hands at your sides (Fig. 82). Rest.

Notes

● You may repeat the exercise once and again later in the day.
● It is *not* necessary to touch the knees. Curl up only to the point where you feel maximum tightness of the abdominal muscles then stop there.

Diagonal Curl-up

1 Lie on your back with your knees bent and the soles of your feet flat on the mat. (Fig. 85). Breathe regularly.

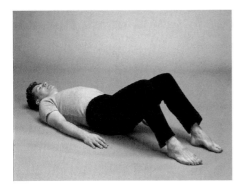

Fig. 85. Diagonal Curl-up – preparation

2 Slowly curl your upper body forwards, reaching with your hands towards the outside of your *right* knee (Fig. 00). Synchronize your movement with regular breathing.
3 Hold this posture only for as long as you are comfortable in it. Keep breathing regularly.

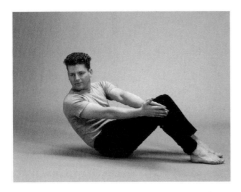

Fig. 86. Diagonal Curl-up – completed, side view

4 Slowly uncurl your body onto the mat to resume your starting position.
5 Repeat the Diagonal Curl-up on the other side. Rest afterwards.

Advanced variation

As you acquire greater strength and become more confident, you may wish to try the Diagonal Curl-up with your arms folded across your chest or clasped behind your neck. In this case, aim your left shoulder toward your right knee as you curl forward, then repeat the curl up, aiming your right shoulder toward your left knee (Figs. 87 and 88).

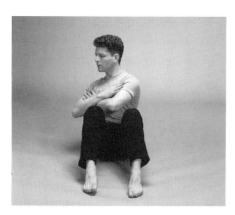

Fig. 87. Diagonal Curl-up – variation, front view

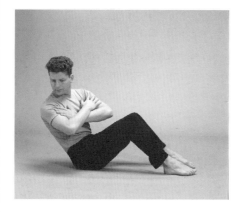

Fig. 88. Diagonal Curl-up – side view

The exercise to follow is advanced. Do it only if you feel ready for it.

1   Sit with your legs bent and the soles of your feet flat on the mat (Fig. 89). Breathe regularly.

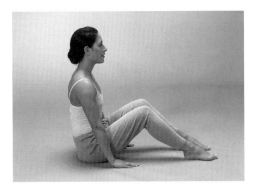

Fig. 89. Angle Balance – sitting up, knees bent

2   Tilt backwards so that you are balancing on your bottom; your feet are off the mat and your knees are closer to your chest. Use your hands to help, if necessary (Fig. 90). Focus your attention on your regular breathing to help you to maintain balance.

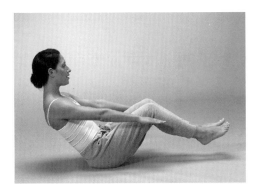

Fig. 90. Angle Balance – feet off ground, tilting back

3   Stretch out your arms so that they are parallel to the mat. Also stretch out your legs (Fig. 91). Keep focused, and adjust the degree of your tilt to help you to keep your balance.

4   Hold the posture as long as you are comfortable in it, while breathing regularly.

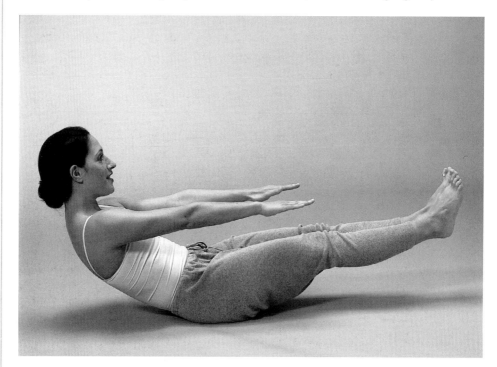

Fig. 91. Angle Balance – completed posture, legs straight

5   Slowly and carefully resume your starting position.
6   Sit or lie down and rest.
7   Repeat the exercise if you wish. Rest afterwards.

Single Leg Raise

1 Lie on your back, with your legs stretched out in front and your arms relaxed beside
   you. Breathe regularly.
2 Bend your left leg and rest the sole of your foot flat on the mat, a comfortable distance
   from your bottom (Fig. 92).

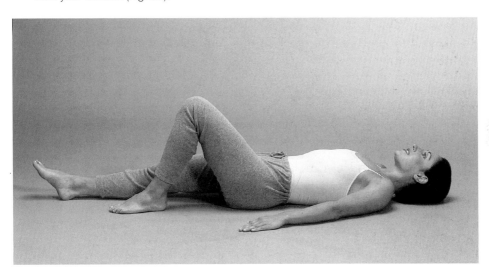

Fig. 92. Leg Raise – left leg bent

3 On an exhalation, while pressing the small of your back (waist) firmly against the mat,
   raise the straight leg slowly and with control, until you feel your lower abdomen tighten.
   If you wish, you may pull your toes towards you, aiming your sole upwards, to give a
   therapeutic stretch to the hamstring muscles at the back of your legs (Fig. 93).
4 Hold the raised-leg posture as long as you feel comfortable doing so. Keep breathing
   regularly.

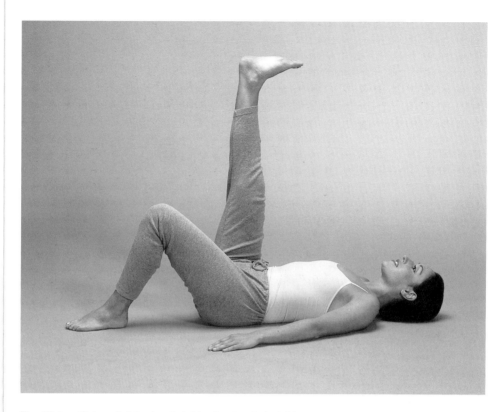

Fig. 93. Leg Raise – left leg bent, right raised and straight

5 Keeping the small of your back pressed firmly to the mat, lower your raised leg slowly and with control, synchronizing the movement with regular breathing.

6 Rest briefly before repeating the exercise with the other leg. Rest afterwards.

Note well

Do *not* raise both legs at once while lying supine (on your back), as this may cause back strain or pain.

The Abdominal Lift

This is an advanced exercise. Do *not* practise it if you have high blood pressure, an ulcer of the stomach or intestine (peptic ulcer), a heart problem or a hiatus hernia (protrusion of the stomach through the diaphragm). Do *not* practise the *Abdominal Lift* if you are pregnant. In any case, *check with your doctor* before attempting to do this exercise.

Practise this exercise on an empty or near-empty stomach; never immediately after having eaten.

1   Stand with your feet about 25 centimetres (10 inches) apart.
2   Bend your knees and turn them slightly outwards, as if preparing to sit.
3   Rest your hands on your thighs. Keep your torso as erect as you comfortably can in this position (Fig. 94). Breathe regularly.

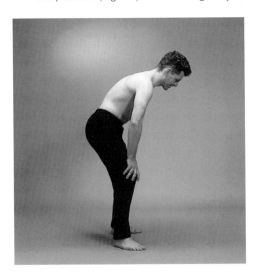

Fig. 94. Abdominal Lift – start position, side view

4   Exhale and with the air still expelled, briskly pull in your abdomen as if to touch your spine with it, and also pull it upwards, towards your ribs (Fig. 95).
5   Hold the abdominal contraction until you feel the urge to inhale.

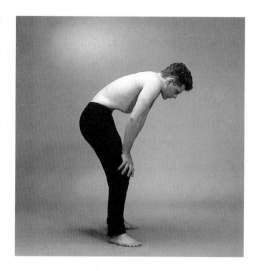

Fig. 95. Abdominal Lift – abdomen held in, side view

6   Inhale and relax your abdomen. Straighten and relax your body and your arms. Resume regular breathing.

You may wish to repeat the exercise once now, and again later in the day if you wish.

To complete the full range of abdominal exercises, please practise the *Half Moon* (Fig. 76, page 88) and the *Spinal Twist* (Figs. 78 and 79, page 89). These two exercises will tone and firm your oblique abdominal muscles which are part of the four-way 'corset' described earlier in this chapter, on pages 89 and 90.

Cooling down

After your exercise session, do remember to cool down. Refer to chapter four, pages 62 to 66 for suggestions.

Strong Legs for a Strong Back

In chapter one, it was pointed out that certain leg muscles were considered secondary supports of the back and that two of them contributed to the balance of the pelvic ring, thus helping to maintain normal spinal curves (*see* page 7). In chapter two, which dealt with posture and body mechanics, emphasis was placed on the use of the leg muscles to help prevent back strain.

It seems to make good sense then, that if we are to 'use the legs to spare the back', they should be strong and flexible and functioning optimally. A brief look at the chief leg muscles involved in preventing backache therefore seems appropriate.

Leg Muscles

Arising at the sides of the lumbar vertebrae, the *psoas* muscle passes along the groin and inserts into the upper thigh bone (femur). The *iliacus* arises from the hipbone and unites with the psoas to insert into the thigh as well. These two (ilio-psoas muscle) flex and rotate the thighs (hip flexors).

The *quadriceps* muscles, four altogether, are situated on the front of the thighs. They arise from the pelvis and the thigh bones and insert into the upper knee cap (patella). They extend, or straighten, the knees.

The *hamstrings*, of which there are three on each leg, run along the back of the thighs, passing from the lower pelvis to insert into the bones of the lower leg (tibia and fibula). They flex the legs and adduct (move towards the middle of the body) and extend the thighs.

The *gluteal muscles*, forming the prominence of the buttocks, help raise the trunk from a stooping to an erect position and tighten the thighs and abduct them (move them away from the body).

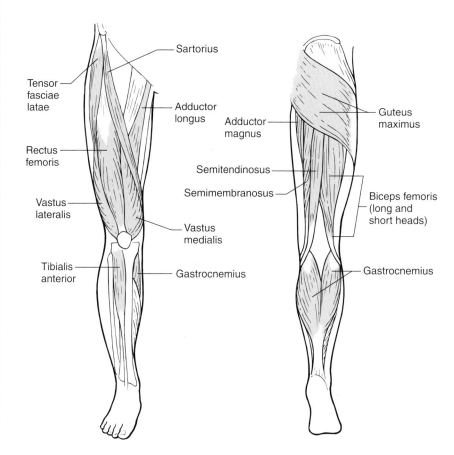

Fig. 96. The leg muscles

Before starting the exercises

Please *check with your doctor* before doing these or any other exercises.

Pregnant women are referred to my book entitled *Easy Pregnancy with Yoga* (*see* bibliography).

Preparing to exercise

Before practising the exercises to follow, be sure to warm up properly (*see* chapter four). Please also review the general instructions also in chapter four, which apply to the practice of all the exercises described in chapters five, six and seven. Here, for quick reference, is a summary of those instructions.

- Wear loose, comfortable clothing which permits you to breathe and stretch easily.
- Practise the exercises on a firm, padded surface, such as a carpeted floor (referred to as the 'mat').
- Concentrate fully on what you are doing. Synchronize your breathing with the body movements.
- Practise the exercises slowly and with complete awareness.
- Once you have completed the exercise, with no strain whatever, maintain the posture for as many seconds as you wish or can with absolute comfort (referred to as 'hold' the position).
- When holding the posture, *do not* hold your breath; keep breathing naturally.
- When you are ready to come out of the posture, do so slowly and with awareness, your movements synchronized with your breathing.
- After completing the exercise, rest briefly before practising another exercise.
- At the end of your exercise session, cool down adequately (*see* chapter four for suggestions).

The Exercises

The Butterfly

1   Sit on your mat with your legs folded inwards and the soles of your feet together. Clasp your hands around your feet and bring the feet comfortably close to your body (Fig. 97). Breathe regularly.

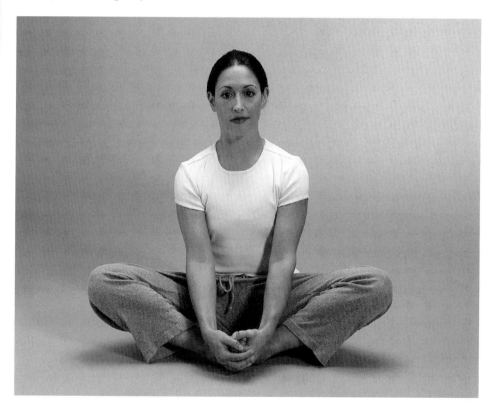

Fig. 97. The Butterfly – knees down

2   Alternately lower your knees (Fig. 98) and raise them, like a butterfly flapping its wings. Do so as many times as you wish, at a slow to moderate pace.

3   Relax your arms and hands and stretch out your legs and rest.

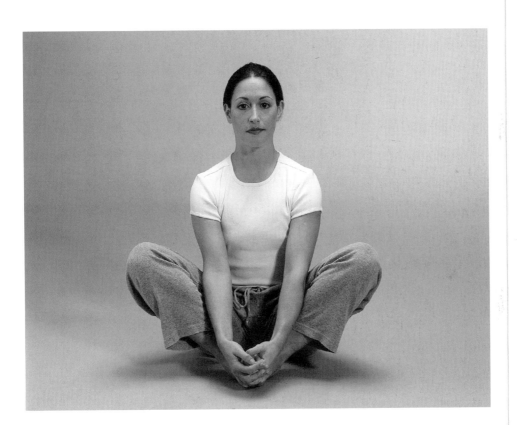

Fig. 98. The Butterfly – knees up

The Butterfly is an excellent warm-up for the legs and hip joints.

For additional exercise for the hip flexor muscles, please practise the knee presses (*see* chapter five, pages 77 to 78).

Balance Posture

1   Stand tall, with your feet comfortably apart and your body weight equally distributed. Relax your arms at your side (Fig. 99). Breathe regularly.

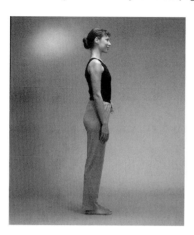

Fig. 99. Balance Posture – start position

2   Shift your weight onto your *left* foot. Focus attention on your breathing to help to keep you steady.
3   Bend your *right* leg. Grasp the ankle with your *right* hand and bring the foot as close to your bottom as you can without straining (Fig. 100).

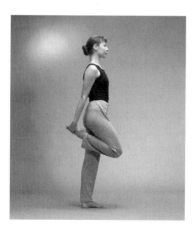

Fig. 100. Balance Posture – right ankle held

4   Raise your *left* arm. Keep it straight and aligned with your ear (Fig. 101).

5   Hold the posture for as long as you comfortably can. Focusing attention on your regular breathing will help you to maintain your balance.

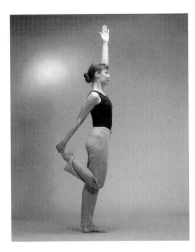

Fig. 101. Balance Posture – complete posture, right ankle held, left arm raised

6   Carefully resume your starting position. Rest.

7   Repeat the exercise, this time standing on your *right* foot and raising your *right* arm. Rest afterwards.

The Balance Posture, sometimes referred to as 'The Quadriceps Stretch', conditions the quadriceps muscles, as the name suggests. It also develops and enhances concentration which, experts say, is a prerequisite for activities such as lifting safely (*see* chapter two, page 24 to 25). I sometimes practise a lying version of the Balance Posture, thus:

Prone Balance Posture

1 Lie prone (face downwards) then turn your head to the side to facilitate breathing. You may place a flat cushion or folded towel under your pelvis to reduce the arch of your lower back. Keep your legs close together or comfortably separated (Fig. 102). Breathe regularly.

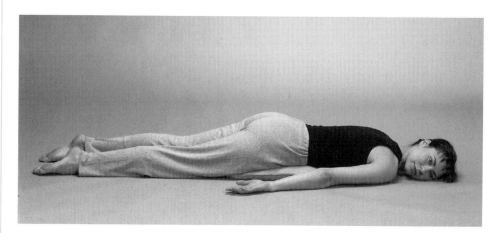

Fig. 102. Prone Balance Posture – start position

2 Bend your legs, bringing your heels towards your bottom (Fig. 103). You should feel a delightful stretch of the thigh muscles as you do so.
3 You may alternately bend and straighten your legs several times, or you may hold the feet in position, as long as this feels comfortable, before resuming your starting position. Rest afterwards.

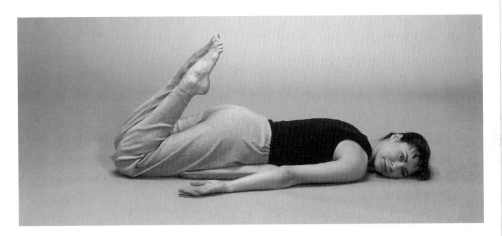

Fig. 103. Prone Balance Posture – complete

Easy variation

For those of you who find it difficult to do the Balance Posture without the aid of a prop, you may hold on with one hand to something stable (such as a post or a sturdy piece of furniture) using the free hand to grasp the foot.

The Dog Stretch

Cautions

Do not practise the Dog Stretch if you suffer from high blood pressure or have a heart condition or any disorder that produces a feeling of light-headedness or dizziness when you hang your head downwards. Check with your doctor.

1   Start in an 'all-fours' posture, on your hands and knees, but position your hands so that your arms slope gently forwards (Fig. 104). Breathe regularly.

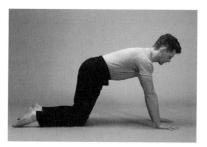

Fig. 104. The Dog Stretch – all-fours, knees on ground

2   Tuck your toes forwards. Rock backwards slightly and raise your knees. Straighten your legs and arms. Look downwards (Fig. 105). Aim your heels towards the mat but do not strain the muscles at the back of your legs (hamstrings).

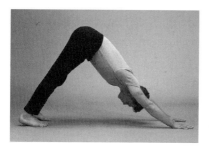

Fig. 105. The Dog Stretch – completed, legs and arms straight

3   Stay in this posture for as long as you are comfortable in it. Keep breathing regularly.

4   Rock forwards gently before returning to your starting position on all-fours. Sit on your heels in the *Japanese Sitting Position* (Fig. 106).

5   Rest in the *Pose of a Child* (Figs. 71 and 72, page 85).

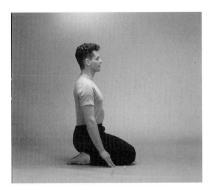

Fig. 106. Dog Stretch – recovery, Japanese Sitting Position

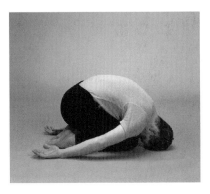

Fig. 107. Dog Stretch – recovery, Pose of a Child

Other exercises which keep the hamstring muscles in good condition include: lunging (chapter two, Fig. 19, page 26) and ankle rotation (chapter four, page 54).

The Half Locust

1   Lie on your abdomen, with your chin touching the mat and your legs slightly separated. Keep your arms straight and beside your body. Make your hands into fists and keep the thumbs down (Fig. 108). Breathe regularly.

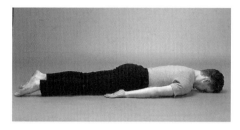

Fig. 108. Half Locust – start position

2   Exhale and slowly and carefully raise one leg, kept straight, as high as you comfortably can. Keep your chin, arms and body pressed to the mat (Fig. 109).
3   Hold the raised-leg posture for as long as you can without straining. Keep breathing regularly.

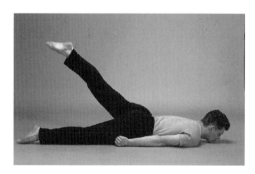

Fig. 109. Half Locust – completed posture, leg raised

4   Lower your leg slowly and with control. Rest.
5   Repeat the exercise with the other leg. Rest.

Following practice of the Half Locust you may try resting in the *Pose of a Child* (Figs. 71 and 72, page 85).

Toe-Finger Posture (Standing)

1   Stand tall, with your body weight equally distributed between your feet and your arms relaxed at your sides (Fig. 110). Breathe regularly.

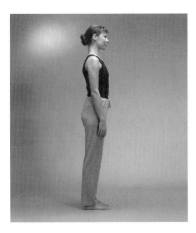

Fig. 110. Toe-Finger Posture – standing

2   Shift your weight onto one foot. Slowly and carefully raise the other foot and bring it towards you (Fig. 111).

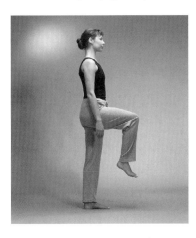

Fig. 111. Toe-Finger Posture – half way

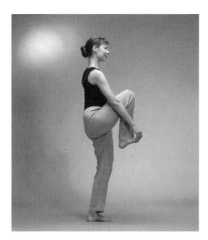

Fig. 112. Toe-Finger Posture – toes held

3 Grasp the toes of the raised foot, using the other arm to help you to maintain balance (Fig. 112). If you focus attention on your regular breathing, it will help you to stay steady.

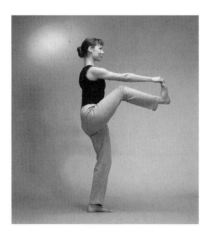

Fig. 113. Toe-Finger Posture – toes held, legs bent

4 Keeping a secure grasp on your toes, carefully straighten the raised leg (Fig. 114). Do not strain the muscles at the back of your leg (hamstrings).

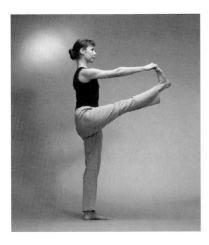

Fig. 114. Toe-Finger Posture – toes held, leg straightened

5   Hold the posture for as long as you can while breathing regularly.
6   Prepare to resume your starting position: slowly bend the raised leg and release your grasp on the toes. Lower your leg and relax your arms. Rest.
7   Repeat the exercise with the other leg. Rest afterwards.

The Toe-Finger Posture (Standing) is not only excellent for improving the tone of your hamstring muscles, but also for strengthening your ankles and your abdomen. In addition, it is superb for developing concentration, which is a prerequisite for the safe performance of activities such as bending, getting up, lifting and shovelling (*see* chapter two, pages 23 to 27).

Variation

The following is a challenging variation of the Toe-Finger Posture (Standing). In addition to the benefits already mentioned, this version of the exercise conditions the inner leg muscles.

1   Stand tall, with your body weight equally distributed between your feet and your arms relaxed at your sides. Breathe regularly.
2   Shift your weight onto one foot. Slowly and carefully raise the other foot and bring it towards you.

3 Grasp the toes of the raised foot, using the other arm to help you to maintain balance.

4 Keeping a secure grasp on your toes, carefully straighten the raised leg. Do not strain the muscles at the back of your leg (hamstrings).

5 Slowly and with control bring the raised leg to the side, as far as you comfortably can. If you focus attention on your regular breathing, it will help to keep you steady.

6 Hold the posture for as long as you comfortably can.

7 Slowly bring the raised leg back to the front and carefully resume your starting position.

8 Repeat the exercise with the other leg. Rest afterwards.

Toe-Finger Posture (Supine)

This is one of my favourite exercises. I find it marvellous for helping to relieve a tired back. It also conditions the leg muscles.

1 Lie on your back (supine) with your legs stretched out in front of you and your arms relaxed at your sides. Breathe regularly.
2 Bend first one leg and then the other, resting your feet flat on the mat.
3 Bring one knee and then the other towards your chest (Fig. 115).

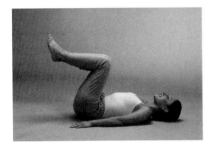

Fig. 115. Toe-Finger Supine – arms down, knees bent

4 Tuck the fingers of your left hand under the toes of your left foot; do the same with the other fingers and toes.
5 Holding the toes securely, carefully straighten your legs (Fig. 116). Do not strain. As your flexibility increases, you will be able to straighten your legs fully.
6 Hold the posture for as long as you comfortably can. Keep breathing regularly.

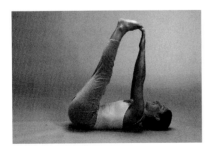

Fig. 116. Toe-Finger Supine – toes held, legs straightened

7 Release the grasp on your toes, bend your legs and, one at a time, place your soles on the mat. Stretch out your legs, rest your arms beside you and relax.

Variation

1 Lie on your back (supine) with your legs stretched out in front of you and your arms relaxed at your sides. Breathe regularly.
2 Bend first one leg and then the other, resting your feet flat on the mat.
3 Bring one knee and then the other towards the chest.
4 Tuck the fingers of your left hand under the toes of your left foot; do the same with the other fingers and toes.
5 Holding the toes securely, carefully straighten your legs. Do not strain.
6 Slowly spread your legs to their comfortable limit (Fig. 117). Keep breathing regularly.

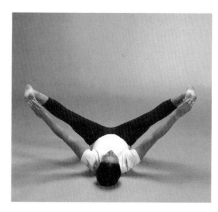

Fig. 117. Toe-Finger Supine – toes held, legs spread

7 Hold the spread-leg posture for as long as you comfortably can.
8 Slowly bring your legs together before resuming your starting position. Rest.

Toe-Finger Posture (Sitting)

This posture is reminiscent of the *Angle Balance* (*see* chapter six, Fig. 91, page 104) and like it is an exercise in concentration.

In addition, the Toe-Finger Posture (Sitting) conditions the leg muscles, particularly the hamstrings and the quadriceps (thigh muscles), which are important in determining the angle of pelvic tilt, and therefore in maintaining good posture (*see* chapter one, page 7).

1   Sit with your legs bent and your soles flat on the mat. Breathe regularly.
2   Bring your knees close to your chest, tilting slightly backwards at the same time, so that your feet are lifted off the mat and you are balancing on your bottom (Fig. 118).

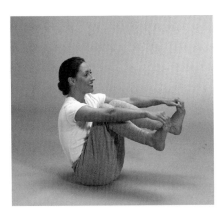

Fig. 118. Toe-Finger Sitting – toes held, knees bent

3   Tuck the fingers of your left hand under the toes of your left foot; do the same with the right fingers and toes. Focus attention on your regular breathing to help you to maintain your balance.
4   Keeping a secure hold on your toes, slowly and carefully straighten your legs (Fig. 119).
5   Hold the posture for as long as you are comfortable in it.

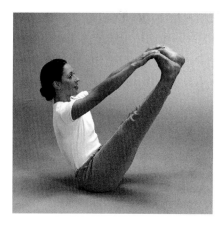

Fig. 119. Toe-Finger Sitting – toes held, legs straight

6   Release the hold on your toes, bring your knees towards you and slowly resume your starting position. Rest.

Cooling down

After completing your exercise session, please remember to cool down. Refer to chapter four for suggestions.

No one can say with certainty why some individuals are more susceptible to back pain than others of similar build and lifestyle. But experts believe that the answer lies partly in the psyche. They base this belief on the observation that suppressed emotions are often at the root of muscular tension which generates pain in the back and head and elsewhere in the body. In short, physical symptoms can be symbolic of underlying psychological problems.

Those who are sceptical of this have only to consider such common reactions as blushing because of embarrassment and sexual arousal at the mere thought of an object of attraction. The mechanisms responsible for these responses may be similar to those producing backache. Indeed, there are many case histories written to illustrate that backache and back pain stem from sources of distress buried in the deep recesses of the mind. One such case is cited by Kenneth Pelletier who tells of a middle-aged cardiologist (heart specialist) with a chronic back problem. His doctor discovered, during therapy, that when the patient was a teenager, he had received a blow from his father. Knocked down windless, the boy huffed and puffed and arched his shoulders backwards, desperately trying to get his wind back. Subsequently, whenever under intense stress, the cardiologist would automatically repeat the rapid breathing and the arching of the back which had brought him relief when he was struck as a boy. Unfortunately these strategies only aggravated his back problem as an adult.

The state of our mind, as experts like Frederick Leboyer have observed, is a reflection of the condition of our back which, though behind us, can influence our mood.

Understanding Pain

The degree of pain experienced is influenced not only by physical factors (such as pressure on nerve endings), but also by religious beliefs, ethnicity and personality. Also playing a part in how we respond to pain stimuli are memory, attention, fear, depression and causes of stress such as job dissatisfaction. All these can intensify and prolong backache and back pain.

Tolerating Pain

In the 1960s, Ronald Melzack, a professor at McGill University, Canada, and Patrick Wall, proposed a theory as to why some individuals seem to tolerate pain better than others. They put forth a spinal 'gate control theory' in which they suggested the existence of a nervous mechanism that, in effect, opens or closes a 'gate' regulating the pain stimuli that reach the brain for interpretation. This mechanism can be affected by certain psychological processes, such as those mentioned earlier: fear, cultural heritage and personality components.

Steven Brena, MD, author of *Yoga and Medicine*, gives an example of how the spinal gate mechanism probably works. Imagine standing in a field or campsite, holding a paper cup of hot beverage. You spill some and burn yourself. You drop the cup and shake your hand around. Now visualize being in your employer's home. In your hand you hold an expensive china cup of tea. Again you burn yourself. This time, however, *you first put the cup down safely, then you shake your hand*. Why are there two different reactions to similar incidents? In the second example when the sensation of burning was relayed to the brain you very quickly *evaluated* the consequences of damaging your employer's rug or breaking the china teacup. The emotional centres in your brain inhibited further sensations of pain until *after* you safely put down the cup and avoided soiling the rug. In the first example, no such inhibition occurred because, upon assessment, you determined that no harm could come to the field or to the paper cup you let fall.

The foregoing is in accord with the spinal gate control theory. Simply put, when the gate is 'open', painful impulses can get through to the brain where they are interpreted as pain.

When the gate is 'closed', however, few or no sensations get through. The spinal gate shuts out, as it were, the entry of sensory inputs.

Closing the gate

How can we close our spinal gate to prevent some of the painful stimuli from reaching the brain? How can we alter our mental evaluation of the hurt?

We can use drugs, such as pain relievers and tranquillizers, to dull emotional responses. These medications, however, can produce side effects such as nausea, high or low blood pressure, dizziness, headache, constipation and other unpleasant symptoms. Alternatively, we can use natural pain control measures.

Natural pain control

According to Dr Brena, everyone has the capacity for limiting or even preventing pain through will-power. Natural pain control methods are largely based on 'closing the gate' to the entry of pain stimuli. Compared with drugs, natural methods have the advantage of producing no deleterious effects. What they do is mobilize the body's own resources to regulate pain and to promote wellbeing. Currently used methods of pain relief include acupuncture, TENS (Transcutaneous Electrical Nerve Stimulation), psychotherapy, biofeedback, hypnosis, the application of heat or cold and massage. These are well-respected, effective pain control approaches. They do, however, require the help of an outside agent, such as a therapist or a machine or gadget. With yoga techniques however, you rely entirely on your own natural resources, which are with you wherever you may be.

Note well

If your pain persists be sure to see a doctor.

Pain relief through yoga

Yoga pain relief techniques work on the following principles:

- trying to prevent painful impulses at the periphery (extremities of the body);
- trying to stop painful impulses as they travel along the spinal cord;
- altering or reducing the perception of, and reaction to, the pain;
- encouraging a greater amount of oxygen to reach body tissues and wash away irritants, and
- attempting to re-educate disused muscles.

The techniques that follow work on these principles.

Meditation

Briefly defined, meditation is doing one thing and only one thing at a time. You focus your attention on one object or activity at a time to the exclusion of everything else.

Chief among the many benefits derived from regular meditation are: the ability to relax while maintaining mental alertness and increased skin resistance which indicates decreased tension and anxiety.

More and more doctors are recommending a period of daily meditation for various health disorders. For your own reassurance, however, *do obtain your doctor's permission* to practise the meditations that follow.

Before starting your meditation:

- select a reasonably quiet place where you won't be interrupted for about half an hour;
- sit comfortably, on a mat or in a chair which adequately supports your spine;
- maintain a well-aligned spinal column and a relaxed body (regular practice of a

relaxation technique, such as the Toe-to-Top relaxation exercise in chapter four (Fig. 41, page 46), will train you to achieve a high degree of relaxation in a short time);

- establish a slow, quiet, regular breathing rhythm, through the nostrils, and
- be completely aware of what you are doing.

Having met all these requirements, you are now ready to begin. Do not be discouraged if you find your mind wandering at first. With regular practice, this will occur less and less, so do persevere.

A basic meditation

1 Sit comfortably with your body relaxed. Pay special attention to your jaw: unclench your teeth and keep your lips together but not compressed. Rest your hands quietly in your lap or on your thighs. Close your eyes. (Fig 120). Breathe regularly.
2 On an exhalation, mentally say the word 'one'.
3 Inhale slowly and smoothly.
4 Mentally say 'one' as you exhale.
5 Continue your repetition of 'one', always on the exhalation.

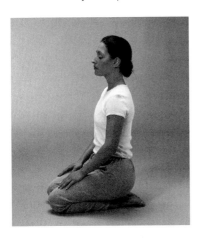

Fig. 120. Meditation – Japanese style

Whenever your attention strays, gently guide it back to your meditation and start again.

Use a word with which you feel completely comfortable. Particularly effective are words compatible with your religious or other beliefs, for example: amen, peace, love, om or shalom.

When you feel the need to end your meditation do so, slowly and with awareness. Never rush. Open your eyes. Leisurely stretch your limbs or massage them gently, or do simple warm-up exercises such as rotating your ankles or shoulders. Take a few deep breaths.

A healing meditation

1   Sit comfortably with your body relaxed. Pay special attention to your jaw: unclench your teeth and keep your lips together but not compressed. Rest your hands quietly in your lap or on your thighs. Close your eyes. (Fig. 121). If you are sitting in a chair with an armrest, rest your hands on those. Breathe regularly.

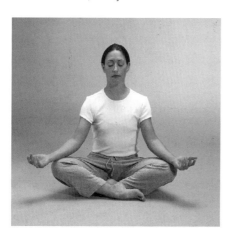

Fig. 121. Meditation – sitting, legs folded

2   As you inhale, visualize an intake of healing energy – perhaps in the form of a soothing light – reaching the affected part, bringing it warmth and relief.

3   As you exhale, visualize the elimination of pain-producing substances through the outgoing breath.

4   Keep your attention focused on the affected part and on your breathing and visualization. If your thoughts stray to unrelated matters, gently guide them back to your meditation.

5   When you feel ready to get up, do so in an unhurried manner: open your eyes, slowly stretch your limbs or do gentle warm-ups – whatever you have the urge to do. Take a few slow, deep breaths.

Variations on a healing meditation

1   Sit or lie comfortably. Relax your jaw and breathe regularly. Close your eyes.

2   Rub your hands together briskly to warm them. Rest them lightly on the affected body part.

3   As you inhale, visualize a soothing stream of water trickling along your arms and through your fingers onto the part that is hurting. Imagine the water with healing properties, lovingly bathing the area.

4   As you exhale, visualize the hurt or pain, perhaps in the form of a mist, drifting away with the outgoing breath.

5   Repeat this exercise as long as you wish, or until you experience relief.

Whenever your attention wanders, gently and patiently redirect it to your breathing and visualization and start again.

Remember to end your meditation slowly and with awareness, having first done some gentle body movements such as ankle rotation or leisurely stretches of your limbs.

Here are other visualizations to try:

• With your mind's eye, picture a soft brush dusting away powder-like deposits that have settled around the joints of your vertebral column, making them stiff and painful. Synchronize the 'brushing' with each inhalation; with each exhalation, imagine the deposits floating away and scattering into the air, never to return.

- Visualize gentle, loving hands applying a soothing, healing balm to the skin over the affected part. As the balm is absorbed through the skin, visualize the affected part becoming less tense, more relaxed, and the hurt disappearing. Synchronize these visualizations with your breathing, which should always be slow and smooth.
- Imagine listening to the dulcet tones of distant music. Feel it at work assuaging your anguish and bringing you comfort.

There are infinite possibilities. The imagery you select should reflect your own natural inclinations and you should be comfortable with it.

Concentration

Concentration, observed the late psychoanalyst Dr Eric Fromm in his well-known work *The Art of Loving*, is rare in our culture. We are inclined to do several things at once: read, listen to the radio or talk while smoking, eating and/or drinking. Yet in order to prevent injury and to be successful in whatever we set out to do, we need to know how to direct and hold attention on one thing or person at a time, regardless of distracting stimuli.

Because of this predisposition for doing several things at once, we often find it difficult to be still. Observe those in any group of which you are a part and you will note how few hands and mouths are at rest. It seems that there is always a compulsion to talk and to move about.

It is only when we learn to be physically and mentally still, however, that we can hope to master the art of concentration. For it is only then that we can give to an activity that undivided attention that is necessary for promoting safety and effectiveness.

It is a misconception that concentrating on something depletes our energy and generates fatigue. When we focus attention on one thing to the exclusion of everything else, it in fact promotes alertness, and the tiredness that follows is healthful rather than enervating.

Since no art can be learned, let alone mastered, without regular practice, here are simple, effective concentration techniques for you to try as part of your daily exercise programme.

(The *Angle Balance*, page 104, the *Balance Posture*, page 115, and the *Toe-Finger Posture*, page 123 also help to develop concentration.)

Candle concentration

For this exercise, place a lighted candle at, or slightly below eye level, on a table or stool, depending on where you are sitting.

1   Look intently at the candle flame, remembering to maintain regular breathing (Fig. 122). If you need to blink, do so.
2   Now close your eyes and retain or recall the image of the flame. If it disappears, don't be anxious. Mentally gaze in the direction of its disappearance and persuade it to come back. Keep breathing regularly.
3   After two minutes, open your eyes. Relax.

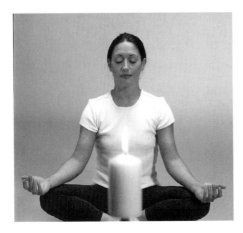

Fig. 122. Candle concentration

With each subsequent exercise session, increase the time spent looking at the flame itself and that spent recalling its image, until your exercise lasts from five to ten minutes.

Variation

Instead of a candle, you may use any other small, pleasing object, such as a flower, a fruit, a design or even a stone on the beach.

Respiratory concentration

1   Sit comfortably. Relax your body. Relax your jaw and breathe regularly. Close your eyes.
2   Inhale slowly, smoothly and as deeply as you can without strain.
3   Exhale slowly and completely without force. At the end of your exhalation, mentally count: 'One thousand, two thousand'.
4   Repeat the exercise: inhalation then exhalation followed by the mental count, as many times as you wish.
5   Open your eyes. Resume regular breathing without counting.

If your attention strays from the breathing and the counting, gently guide it back and start again.

This exercise helps to counteract anxiety, which tends to aggravate pain.

Concentration on sound

1   Sit comfortably. Relax your jaw. Relax the rest of your body. Close your eyes. Breathe regularly.
2   Inhale slowly, smoothly and as deeply as you can without strain.
3   As you exhale slowly and smoothly, make a steady humming sound, like that of a bee. Let the humming last as long as the exhalation does. Do not strain.
4   Repeat inhalation followed by exhalation with humming as many times as you wish. Try to become totally immersed in the sound.
5   Open your eyes and resume regular breathing, without the humming.

If your attention wanders, gently redirect it to your exercise and start again.

Breathing Exercises

Earlier in this chapter (page 132), I outlined principles on which yoga pain-relief techniques work. The visualization exercises described are useful in helping to alter or reduce the perception of, and reaction to, any discomfort or pain felt. They help to prevent painful stimuli from reaching the brain.

The breathing exercises which follow are also based on these principles. In addition, they encourage a better oxygen supply to reach body tissues to wash away irritants contributing to discomfort and pain. They also help to re-educate the muscles involved in the breathing process, chiefly the diaphragm, which is situated between the chest and the abdomen.

Prerequisites for effective breathing

1   A naturally erect position of the vertebral column (spine), with the ribcage relaxed so as to avoid compression of the lungs and other major organs in the chest (heart and large blood vessels).
2   A slow, steady, deep inhalation, first using the diaphragm somewhat as a suction pump, and then expanding the ribcage with the help of the chest muscles.
3   A slow, steady exhalation, using mainly the diaphragm in reverse action as a sort of a squeezing pump.
4   A regular breathing rhythm.
5   Unless otherwise specified, breathe through your nostrils, with your mouth closed, so that the air may be warmed and moistened before entry into the lungs.
6   A relaxed body. Pay special attention to the jaw, face and hands.

After breathing slowly and deeply, the oxygenation of the blood is known to improve. This means better nourishment of body tissues, and improved elimination of waste products which are injurious to health.

Diaphragmatic breathing

1 Lie on your back, with your legs outstretched in front and comfortably separated. Bend your arms and rest the palms of your hands flat on your abdomen so that the tips of the middle fingers meet above your navel. Close your eyes.

2 Begin with a slow, smooth inhalation through the nostrils, making it as deep as possible without incurring discomfort. Focus your attention on the muscular movements of your chest and abdomen: your ribcage expands and your abdomen rises. The fingers separate.

3 Exhale slowly and smoothly through the nostrils, again focusing attention on the chest and abdomen: the ribcage relaxes and the abdomen flattens. The middle fingers again touch in midline.

4 Repeat the exercise: inhalation followed by exhalation as many times as you wish, in smooth succession.

5 Relax your arms and hands at your sides. Breathe regularly.

Variation

Instead of having your legs stretched out in front, you may bend them, placing the feet flat on the surface on which you are lying, a comfortable distance from your bottom. I like positioning my legs so that my knees lean against each other and my feet are apart.

The Alternate Nostril Breath

Here is a very soothing breathing exercise. It helps to allay anxiety which worsens physical discomforts and pain. It is also an effective antidote for sleeplessness, which many people who have back problems experience.

1   Sit with your spine held naturally erect and supported if necessary. Relax your body. Relax your jaw and breathe regularly.
2   Rest your left hand quietly in your lap or on your knee, or on the armrest of a chair.
3   Arrange the fingers on your right hand as follows: fold the two middle fingers towards your palm (or you may rest them lightly on the bridge of your nose). You will use your thumb to close your right nostril once the exercise is in progress, and your ring finger (or ring and little fingers) to close your left nostril (Fig. 123).

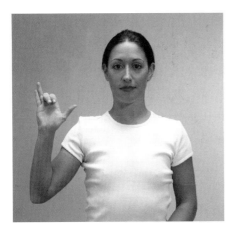

Fig. 123. Alternate Nostril Breathing – start position

4   Close your eyes and begin: close your right nostril and inhale slowly, smoothly and as deeply as you can without strain through your left nostril (Figs. 124 and 125).
5   Close your left nostril and release closure of your right. Exhale.
6   Inhale through your right nostril.
7   Close your right nostril, release closure of your left and exhale.

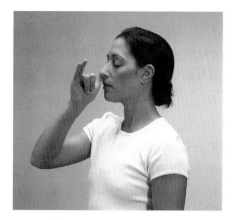

Fig. 124. Alternate Nostril Breathing – side view

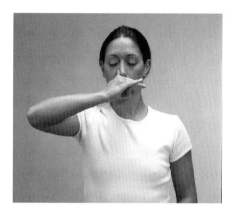

Fig. 125. Alternate Nostril Breathing – front view

This completes one 'round' of Alternative Nostril Breathing. Do a few more rounds to start with. When you become familiar with the technique and comfortable with it, increase the duration of your practice.

8   Relax your right arm and hand. Open your eyes. Resume regular breathing.

All-Body Relaxation

The following exercise is a variation of the *Top-to-Toe Relaxation (Savasana),* described in chapter four (Fig. 41, page 66). In this version, however, you dispense with the alternate tightening and relaxation of various muscles. Breathe regularly throughout the exercise.

You can practise this all-body relaxation technique in a variety of places: on your exercise mat, in an easy chair, on your bed or even while sitting in a doctor's or dentist's waiting-room. Close your eyes if it is safe and convenient to do so, or keep them open. Here's how to do it.

1   Start with your feet, mentally isolating them from the rest of the body. Give them silent suggestion to let go of their tightness and to relax. For instance, you may say in your mind: 'Toes relax. Feet relax'. Try to sense a lessening of tension.
2   Next focus your attention on your lower legs. Give them silent suggestion to let go of their tension. Try to be aware of your calf muscles relaxing.
3   Move upwards to the thighs. Give them positive mental suggestion to release their tightness. Sense their relaxation.
4   Concentrate next on your abdominal muscles. As you inhale, be conscious of a gentle rising of your abdomen. As you exhale, let your abdomen relax. Do this a few times.
5   Continue in this manner, mentally isolating various body parts, and giving each a silent instruction to give up its tension and to relax. The following sequence is suggested:

From your abdomen move upwards to your ribcage. As you inhale, note how your chest expands and note how it relaxes as you exhale. Repeat this a few times.

Proceed to your back: your buttocks, the small of your back and your upper back between your shoulderblades.

Attend next to your hands, arms and shoulders. Follow this with relaxing your neck, both back and front.

Finish with your scalp muscle, which runs from above your eyebrows to the back of your head; unclench your teeth to relax your jaw; relax your lips, tongue, cheeks, forehead and eyes.

End your attention fully focused on your breathing. Each time you inhale, imagine filling your being with positive forces such as gratitude, hope and love. Each time you exhale, visualize sending away negative influences such as resentment, anger and hopelessness, or unwanted feelings such as anxiety or pain. With each exhalation also, let your body sink more deeply into the surface on which you are lying or sitting. Surrender yourself completely to the calm that begins to envelop you.

Come out of your state of deep relaxation slowly and with awareness. Move your head gently from side to side, leisurely stretch your limbs or do whatever you have the urge to do or whatever you conveniently can. Remember to get up carefully so as not to strain your back.

Sleeping for Backache Relief

Every year, tons of sleeping pills are consumed by thousands of individuals seeking relief from the inability to enjoy a good night's sleep. Why is it that some people seem to function well with a mere four hours of sleep, while other wake up tired and aching after eight hours in bed?

The causes of insomnia, or habitual sleeplessness, fall roughly under two headings: non-physical causes, as seen in anxiety states, and physical, as in bodily discomfort or pain, such as backache. Often, however, people say they have insomnia because of long-term dissatisfaction with the duration and/or the quality of sleep. Some individuals become obsessed with the idea that they must have eight hours of sleep each night. If they miss a half-hour, they view it as a disaster. The fact is that some people need only five or six hours' sleep at night to function optimally the next day. Moreover, as we grow older, we tend to need less sleep than when we were younger.

The first remedy for sleeplessness is to determine the cause or causes of it. Here are 14 questions to ask yourself to help you to pinpoint what's at the root of your inability to have a restful night's sleep:

1 What causes you to awaken during the night (for example, pain, hunger, having to go to the toilet)?

2 Is your insomnia a possible side effect of medication you are taking?

3 Do you take a nap in the evening after supper?

4 Do you habitually drink alcoholic beverages in the evening to help you to fall asleep?

5 Do you drink tea, coffee or other beverages containing caffeine before going to sleep?

6 Do you eat a large meal shortly before going to sleep?

7 Do you smoke before going to sleep?

8 Do you exercise vigorously before going to sleep?

9 Do you take a hot shower or bath before going to bed for the night?

10 Do you read exciting stories or watch stimulating television shows before going to bed?

11 Are your bed and bedclothes absolutely comfortable?

12 Is your room temperature too hot or too cold?

13 Do you often go to bed with unresolved problems on your mind?

14 Have you discussed your sleep problems with a health professional?

The answers to the foregoing questions should enable you to gain some insight into why you are not enjoying a refreshing night's sleep. A check-up with your doctor is also a good idea, to help to rule out any physical causes at the root of the problem.

Remedies for sleeplessness

Orthodox medical treatments for insomnia and other forms of sleeplessness rely heavily on medications. These drugs, however, are not without unpleasant side effects. Certain hypnotic agents can, in fact, disturb the normal sleep cycle and produce drowsiness, confusion and memory loss. Long-term use of pharmaceutical sleep aids simply masks the problem; it does not solve it.

The following, by contrast, are natural measures to promote sound sleep. They do not produce the adverse reactions some drugs do.

Sleep serves two primary functions: to restore energy and to help the body to regulate and synchronize itself. Studies show that people deprived of sleep manifest various disturbing symptoms, including psychotic behaviour.

With specific reference to the health of the spine, I mentioned in chapter one (page 2), that when we are sleeping or resting, the intervertebral discs suck in water and other nutrients. This compensates for the squeezing out of fluids from the discs when we are awake and active.

Recipe for a Good Night's Sleep

The following are some of the main ingredients necessary for a night of sound, refreshing sleep.

Pre-sleep activities

Mild exercise after supper can promote sound sleep, whereas vigorous exercise may prove too stimulating. All the exercises in chapter four on pages 45 to 46 are suitable to practise at night before going to sleep. The breathing exercises are also appropriate, as well as the all-body relaxation technique described in this chapter.

A warm (*not* hot) bath is relaxing and some people find it sleep-inducing. The water should be between 35°C and 38°C (95°F to 100°F). *See also* the section on herbal baths later in this chapter, page 151.

It is not a good idea to take a nap in the evening, as it may interfere with your night's sleep. Avoid reading stimulating literature or watching disturbing television shows if you have observed that they detract from the quality of your night's sleep.

As you prepare to sleep, try to turn your thoughts away from unpleasant matters. Consciously try to focus attention on positive experiences instead. Practise the *Top-to-top relaxation* exercise described in chapter four, pages 65 to 66, and towards the end of it spend a few minutes visualizing a peaceful scene or recalling an experience that brought you joy and contentment. You may also practise *Diaphragmatic Breathing* (*see* page 140) or the *Alternate Nostril Breath* (*see* page 141) following the *Top-to-top relaxation*.

Food, drink and tobacco

Make your last meal of the day a light and easily digested one. If you find that you can't sleep because you are hungry, place a light snack at your bedside, such as cereal or a thermos of warm milk, so you don't have to go to the kitchen to prepare it. (The calcium in the milk, in addition to being sleep promoting, is good for your bones, and the amino acid tryptophan, which it also contains, is a known soporific.) Two or three calcium tablets taken with the warm milk is another good relaxant, especially if you have a calcium deficiency. *Check with your doctor or nutrition counsellor.*

Avoid drinking alcoholic beverages shortly before bedtime, since they detract from the quality of sleep. Also, avoid stimulants such as tea, coffee, cocoa and cola drinks at night.

Healing, ventilation, noise and light

Before going to bed for the night, check that the room temperature is comfortable. Some people find that a somewhat cool temperature is more conducive to restful slumber than one which is too warm.

If the room is stuffy, it may cause you to wake up in the morning feeling less than refreshed. If the weather is suitable, try sleeping with a window open.

Heavy curtains help to darken a room and keep out disturbing sounds. Ticking clocks should be removed if they bother you, and rattling doors and windows should be fixed.

Bed and bedding

The bed on which you habitually sleep should be sufficiently firm to give your body good support without causing stiffness, aches or other forms of discomfort. If your mattress sags, it will subject major muscles and ligaments to strain and produce tension build-up.

Whereas some people are high in their praise of waterbeds, others are sceptical of them. Do experiment to find out what is best for you.

If you have neck problems, consider using an improvised neck collar: roll a small towel into a sausage shape and place it around your neck. This will give your head support and prevent it from rolling.

Keep bedclothes to a minimum. Heavy bedding may impede the proper circulation of blood.

Some individuals find that the position of the bed makes a difference to the quality of their sleep. Sleeping in a north-to-south position, they find, is more conducive to restful slumber and a feeling of vitality the next day than when they sleep in an east-to-west position. This is probably because the body, being a magnetic field, better harmonizes with the earth's magnetic current when placed in the former position.

If you are very sensitive and suffer from insomnia, and you have tried everything you can think of to remedy the difficulty without success, you may wish to put the above suggestion to the test. You certainly have nothing to lose and you may be delightfully surprised.

Postures for sleeping and relaxing

All yoga postures and breathing and meditation exercises have the potential for counteracting tension and fatigue, promoting rest and replenishing energy. Some, however, aim specifically at body-mind relaxation and sleep of the best quality. The *Top-to-toe Relaxation (Savasana)* in chapter four, pages 65 to 66 is perhaps unsurpassed. It is usually practised in a supine position, that is, lying on the back, as illustrated in Fig. 41, page 66.

A variation of this posture, which may be practised in an easy chair, was described earlier in this chapter (the *All-Body Relaxation*, on page 143).

Another yoga relaxation posture, the *Stick Posture*, was described in chapter four, page 63 as well. Instead of using it as an all-body stretch, you may simply rest in the position described: lie at full length on your back, with your arms extended about your head, and the palms of the hands turned upwards. Separate your legs for maximum comfort. Breathe slowly and rhythmically.

At the slightest suggestion of strain on the lower back, modify the position, thus: bend your legs, place the soles of the feet flat on the surface on which you are lying, a comfortable distance from your bottom, and lean one knee against the other. Experiment until you find the position that's best for you.

The *Crocodile Posture* (also called the Dolphin Posture) is done lying face downwards, stretched out at full length, somewhat like a prone version of the Stick Posture. You may adjust your head for ease of breathing, and your arms and legs for maximum comfort. Turn the palms of your hands downwards. Remember to practise slow, rhythmic breathing.

Note

In chapter two, page 21, I mentioned that, generally, it is not a good idea to lie prone; certainly not for long periods. Some people, however, find the face downwards position relaxing when practised for short periods.

When lying prone, therefore, it's a good idea to place a thin cushion or folded towel under your hips, to prevent accentuation of the arch of the lower spine and strain of the back muscles.

A variation of the Crocodile Posture is to position your arms alongside your body, rather than stretched out ahead. This then becomes somewhat of a prone equivalent of *Savasana* (Fig. 41, page 66). Do adjust your head position for comfort and ease of breathing.

Side Relaxation Posture

This posture is reminiscent of the lying position illustrated in Fig. 16, in chapter two, page 22. In this instance, however, there are modifications: if you lie on your left side, for instance, you fold your left arm and rest your head on your left palm. Your right leg rests on top of the left, both slightly bent for maximum comfort. The right arm rests at the right side of the body, either on the right thigh or placed beside the left arm. Place a pillow between your legs, if you wish.

Reverse the instructions if you lie on your right side. Also, remember to keep the spine well aligned and to breathe slowly and rhythmically.

The foregoing postures are suitable for brief periods of relaxation. For longer periods of rest and sleep, the lying positions described in chapter two (Figs. 15 and 16) may be more appropriate. Do experiment with the various positions to find those that are best for you.

Herbal remedies

Infusions of sedative herbs such as catmint, camomile flowers, dill, hops, lime blossom, melitot, passion flower, sage and valerian will help to calm you down and promote a pleasant drowsiness.

Make the infusion as you would brew ordinary tea, generally using one teaspoon of the herb to a cup of water. Drink a cupful of the beverage shortly before going to bed. You may sweeten the drink with a little unpasteurized honey, if you wish.

Another herbal tea you can try is this: add a pinch of lime flowers, a pinch of marjoram and a pinch of vervain to a cupful of hot water. Let the herbs infuse for a few minutes. Strain the tea and sip it slowly, sweetened or unsweetened.

Hops pillows

Hops pillows are an old standby for problem sleepers. To make a pillow, sew together two squares of fabric (the measurements depend on the size of pillow you wish; a small one is adequate).

Fill the pillow with hops cones. If you find the scent overpowering, add other herbs such as lavender or rose petals, with emphasis on the hops.

As you breathe in the scent of the hops, you will become drowsy and fall asleep.

Herbal baths

A warm bath containing an infusion of hops (and other herbs if you wish) taken shortly before slipping into a warm bed will promote recuperative sleep.

A bath containing essential oils, such as those from hops, orange blossom and meadowsweet can also be wonderfully relaxing.

It is often the fear of insomnia rather than the sleeplessness itself that produces the deleterious effects of a poor night's rest. Don't let sleep obsess you to the point where if you miss an hour or half an hour of it, you regard it as a calamity.

Follow the suggestions in this chapter and anything else you consider useful to promote adequate sleep. If everything tried is to no avail, however, *seek a doctor's advice*. If he or she prescribes medication, take it but continue practising the relaxation techniques in this book.

Using Your Head to Save Your Back

Stress has become a household word. It is something without which we cannot live. It is what enables some individuals to achieve great things. When stress is continuous and unrelieved, however, it becomes a destructive force. It produces unnecessary tension which can spread and cause discomfort, aches and pain. It can drain our energy and make us feel exhausted. Stress detracts from the joy of living.

What is stress?

Stress occurs when the demands of our internal or external environment, or both, tax or overwhelm our personal resources for dealing with them.

Effects of stress

Stress brings about undesirable changes in the structure and function of body tissues. These changes are largely responses to hormones secreted by glands located above the kidneys (the adrenal glands). They include:

- increased pulse rate;
- elevated blood pressure;
- faster rate of breathing;
- temporary impairment of digestion;
- withdrawal of minerals from bones;
- mobilization of fat from storage deposits;
- retention of an abnormal amount of salt in the body.

Stressors

A stressor is something that generates stress. It may be an event, a circumstance or some other agent. How it affects you depends essentially on how you perceive it. One person may regard a certain incident as comical and laugh about it. Another individual may look at the same occurrence and be offended or distressed by it, and for the latter individual that occurrence may be stressful.

Types of stressors

Stressors can take the form of everyday irritations in our relationship with others: spouse, children, acquaintances and co-workers. Some stressors are more short-term yet more powerful – like a bereavement. All these stressors take a toll on our system and all have the potential to produce chronic problems, to deplete our energy and to undermine our health.

Notorious stressors include apprehension, anxiety, fear, guilt, conflict, regret and uncertainty. These are all negative emotions that eventually compromise our health.

Another well-recognized stressor is having too many life changes occur in too short a period of time, for instance, losing one's job, moving house, starting a new career and starting a new relationship, all in the same year. Experts predict that this increases the risk of a serious illness or accident and I have seen their prediction come to pass again and again.

Control is the secret

Stressors lose their impact when they cease to deprive you of a sense of control. Once you learn to view an event, circumstance or other potential stressor as something over which you do have a measure of control, and which is not going to last forever, you have made an important first step in effective stress management.

Strategies for effective stress control

Information is the first step towards effective stress management. Be informed, so as to equip yourself to combat harmful stressors.

Keeping fit is an essential second step towards effective stress control. All the exercises – physical, breathing, and meditative – in this book will contribute to your keeping fit. In addition, the nutrition information in chapter three will be useful to help you to provide your body with the correct nutritive material for peak fitness.

The third positive step towards intelligent stress control is to establish and maintain a reliable emotional support system. This could be a trusted, dependable friend or group of friends or a professional counsellor with whom you have a good rapport. A good support system will provide you with encouragement when you feel discouraged and will furnish you with a safe, healthy outlet for feelings that need to be expressed rather than suppressed. A good support system will, moreover, reinforce positive feelings and promote a sense of self-worth and self-confidence, which are often destroyed when you feel despondent. Again and again, research has shown that stifling emotions results in hurt to oneself rather than to others.

To complement the three foregoing main stress management strategies, here are others suggested by various experts on stress:

- During the first few unpleasant moments of a stressful situation try this: smile inwardly and also with your eyes and mouth to reduce facial tension. Take a smooth, slow, deep breath in, and then exhale steadily while letting go of tightness from your jaw, tongue and shoulders. Mentally tell yourself that you are calm, alert and in control.
- Learn to identify and to anticipate both internal and external sources of stress.
- Learn to recognize symptoms of stress such as a racing heartbeat or heart palpitations, irritability, anxiety, diarrhoea, tight jaw and a tense back.
- Regularly practise a relaxation technique you enjoy and find effective. I have described some in detail earlier in this chapter, and also in chapter four, pages 63 to 66. Regular practice of a relaxation technique will provide you with a break from routine activities and help you to replenish your energy supplies. It will help to reduce the impact of stressful stimuli and allow you time to recover. It will enable you to become more in touch with yourself and thus better able to recognize symptoms of stress.
- Have some fun. Psychologists and psychiatrists agree that play is very important for wellbeing. Balance work with a hobby or sport you enjoy. Avoid bringing to your recreation the spirit of competition or the compulsion to win. Play for pleasure.
- Delegate chores so that you are not overburdened. Learn to say 'no' without feeling

guilty when this is appropriate. This prevents overcommitment. Learn how to be assertive yet gracious.

- Learn to laugh. Laughter is one of the best medicines you can take and it has no adverse effects.
- Practise not giving to others the power to make you react before you are fully ready to act. (Review the first of the above stress management suggestions.)

Stress at work

Effective time management is an essential part of stress management. Aches and pain in the neck and back are sometimes a manifestation of continual hard mental and/or physical work without the balancing effects of adequate rest and relaxation, regular exercise and adequate nutrition. Backache and related symptoms are sometimes a consequence of working hard rather than working intelligently.

Here are some tips from experts on making the best of available time so you don't become over-stressed wondering how you're going to find time to do all you have and want to do:

- Keep fit. Back problems, lack of energy and illness result in poor work performance and absenteeism.
- Reduce clutter. When in doubt, throw it out! Reduce paper waste; use the telephone when you can. If you haven't used an item for years, consider giving it to a charitable organization or discard it.
- Shorten tea and coffee breaks. Use such breaks for rest from routine chores and for refreshment; not for prolonged socializing. Try taking a 'yoga break' and practising some of the local relaxation techniques described in chapter four. You can also practise breathing exercises during your breaks.
- Profit from travel time. If you have to travel to and from your place of work, find ways to use the time constructively. Listen to a cassette to help you to improve skills related to your work or to further inform you about ways of coping with stress. Practise 'en route' exercises, such as described in chapter nine, pages 165 to 166.
- Plan your work. Management efficiency experts emphasize that time spent planning is not wasted. Planning, in fact, saves time in the long term.

- Learn to concentrate. Inability to concentrate results in time wasted through having to backtrack and undo or re-do projects. Inability to concentrate can also lead to injury and accidents. Try practising, on a regular basis, the concentration techniques described earlier in this chapter, on pages 136 to 138.

- Control interruptions. Learn to protect your prime time. Unplug your telephone or let your answering machine take your calls. Catch up on work when others are on their breaks. It's not time itself that's significant to the successful completion of a project; it's the amount of *uninterrupted* time.

- Don't procrastinate. Explore why you tend to procrastinate; there may be underlying psychological reasons. Ask yourself why you're putting off that job. Ask what benefits you would derive if you were to tackle it promptly and finish it. The answer may help you to overcome the delays.

- Avoid perfectionism. It's impossible to achieve perfection, in most cases, and it's frustrating to attempt to do so. Frustration is a stressor. Aim instead for excellence of effort and performance.

- Shorten telephone calls. Most phone calls, incoming and outgoing, can be shortened without disaster. Try this: time all calls for the next week or so. Record their length. Try ways of shortening them.

- Cut down on television viewing. Unless a programme entertains or enlightens you, consider not watching it. Read instead, or play word games (or other games) in which family members can participate. The time spent with family will enhance interpersonal relationships and contribute to the support system mentioned earlier in this chapter, in the section on stress management, on pages 153 to 155.

- Don't be a workaholic. It takes intelligence and discernment to distinguish between activities that bring positive results and those that simply help pass the time away. The antidote for workaholism is not to work harder, but to be more organized.

- Don't be too house proud. Keep the home reasonably clean and tidy. Practise 'minimal maintenance'. Rather than have an exhausting major clean-up once a month, for example, clean one room today, another tomorrow and another the next day. Enlist help from family members. Delegate chores.

- Relax! Backache and back pain and associated fatigue are prime timewasters. Incorporate simple relaxation techniques into your work day. The warm-ups in chapter four and the breathing exercises in this chapter are examples of suitable techniques you can weave into daily schedules.

Other Pain Control Measures

The physical exercises, posture awareness techniques and the breathing, concentration and relaxation exercises already discussed are the most important elements in caring for your back and helping to prevent problems. There are, however, additional pain-relief measures which can be helpful. They alleviate symptoms but they do not change poor posture habits or help you to cope with stress. Please check with your doctor before using any of them as adjuncts to natural pain-management methods.

TENS (Transcutaneous Electric Nerve Stimulation)

Electrical therapy for pain relief is not a new concept: the ancient Greeks and Egyptians used electric eels, catfish and torpedo rays to produce analgesia. But electrotherapy was not widely accepted until Melzack and Wall formulated the gate control theory of pain (page 130).

TENS is a convenient non-addictive type of pain therapy which is easy to learn and which can be used in the course of daily activities. Several companies now produce pocket-size battery-operated TENS devices and these can be obtained through surgical supplies stores.

An electrical current is sent into the muscles through electrodes which are taped to the skin and connected to a small power source which can be worn on a belt. The current blocks the transmission of pain to the brain and so helps to break the cycle in which muscle spasm produces pain, which in turn produces further muscle spasm.

TENS seems to be contraindicated only for those persons wearing certain cardiac (heart) pacemakers. The only side effect noted is occasional skin irritation in persons who are allergic to adhesive tape. This can be minimized, however, by using hypoallergenic electrodes, by slightly altering the position of the electrodes, or by using a different conductive gel.

Heat and cold

Temperature changes through the application of heat or cold lead to the relaxation of muscles in areas where the heat or cold is applied.

Local application of heat causes blood vessels in the area to widen (vasodilation). Immediately after the heat is applied, nerve impulses diminish in number, and this causes the muscles to relax.

The application of cold produces a pattern of vasoconstriction (blood vessels tightening) followed by vasodilation. The decreased initial blood flow is accompanied by reduced conduction of nerve impulses and the relaxation of muscles. This alternating pattern helps to remove waste products from the tissues and reduce swelling.

Some people find relief from heat, whereas others prefer ice. If you use a hot-water bottle, be sure that it is covered so as to avoid burns. If you use a heating-pad, be sure that it has an automatic shut-off to avoid burns if you should fall asleep.

Ice should be applied for only about 20 minutes per hour.

NSAIDs (Non-steroidal Anti-inflammatory Drugs)

These are a class of drugs developed to treat arthritis. They are effective in treating a number of mild to moderate pains of non-arthritic origin. NSAIDs decrease inflammation, but their pain-relieving properties are mostly attributed to their ability to block prostaglandin synthesis. (Prostaglandins are highly reactive short-lived molecules. Their main action is that of local messengers which regulate the activity of tissues in which they are formed. Aspirin is one of the oldest NSAIDs and one of the most widely used.)

The most common problem associated with these drugs is gastrointestinal upset (referring to the stomach and intestines) and possibly also bleeding.

Nonanalgestic pain relievers

A number of other drugs, not typically associated with pain relievers, are sometimes used for certain types of pain. Tricyclic antidepressants such as amitriptyline (Elavil) are very effective when used for neuropathic pain (pertaining to any disease of the nerves). They can be taken once a day at bedtime, so that the drowsiness associated with them may promote sleep.

Muscle relaxants may provide short-term relief if the pain is due partially to muscle spasm. The most effective muscle relaxants are tranquillizers, but they tend to make you drowsy and are also potentially addictive.

Massage

Gentle massage is a form of cutaneous stimulation (stimulating the skin to relieve pain). A proper massage not only blocks the perception of pain impulses, but also helps to relax muscle tension and spasm which intensify pain.

Massage improves blood circulation and the elimination of waste products. It also enhances the effects of other pain-relief measures.

Special Needs – Pregnancy, Sports, Driving and More

In the introduction to this book I remarked that almost everyone will experience some form of backache or pain or related symptom at some time. There are those of us, however, who are more susceptible to back problems because of the type of occupation in which we're regularly engaged, or sport in which we habitually participate.

It would be impossible to include all activities and conditions that put the back at risk. I have, however, selected some I consider particularly noteworthy and these follow.

Back Talk for Sportspeople

Although the spine is not the most frequently injured part of the body in athletes, epidemiologic studies indicate that it sustains a high proportion of the most serious injuries.

The spine provides the support and balance essential to stance and to the active motions of sports, such as running, jumping and kicking.

Sports most often associated with spinal injury include gymnastics, football, racquet sports, diving, horseback riding, trampolining and rugby. Racquet sports such as tennis and squash apply substantial torque and rotational force to the spine. In golf, the twisting motion accompanying the drive is the risky part of the sport, since it can damage the intervertebral discs and the facet joints. These motions are often complex and involve sudden changes in direction.

As the spine ages, injuries tend to be of a more chronic and degenerative nature, and it becomes more important than before to pay special attention to any existing weakness, contracture or imbalance, as well as to one's endurance. Many older people who go skiing, for example, have some form of degenerative bone disorder, such as osteoporosis. If you are one of these individuals, you should take extreme care since breaks will occur far more easily than if you were younger.

Even young athletes are not exempt from back problems. Those with weak abdominals and tight hamstrings may be candidates for spinal injuries. Chapter six offers effective exercises for improving abdominal muscle tone, while chapter seven is devoted to exercises for the leg muscles.

There is no doubt whatever that those who are in peak physical condition are less liable to sustain injuries during sporting activities than those who are not.

Occasional athletes usually comprise the bulk of sports participants. These athletes spend most of the week in sedentary occupations and play tennis or go horseback riding on weekends. For both men and women in this group, conditioning is particularly important. In addition, a period of training is essential to develop the muscles used in the particular sport engaged in, and to maintain that muscular development. You must have a warm-up period before participating in your chosen sport (*see* chapter four, pages 45 to 6) and your body weight should be controlled (review chapter three, pages 29 to 43).

If you are recovering from a spinal injury, it is very important to refrain from activities that subject the spine to torque and rotational force (such as racquet sports) until an orthopaedic physician has assessed the damage and given you permission to resume them. Rehabilitation exercise such as walking, cycling and swimming is often recommended during the convalescent period.

Low back pain in athletes

About three out of five athletes who experience low back pain state that their pain appears after they have participated in a sport or similar activity. Robin McKenzie, an internationally known consultant physiotherapist, has remarked that the true cause of pain in many of these individuals is the adoption of a slouched position following a thorough exercising of the joints involved.

During strenuous exercise, the joints of the spine are moved vigorously in many directions over a long period of time. This causes thorough stretching in all directions of the soft tissues surrounding the joints. Moreover, the fluid gel content of the spinal discs (*see* chapter one, page 2 to 3) is loosened and it would appear that distortion or displacement can occur if exercised joints are subsequently placed in an extreme posture, such as collapsing in a heap or slouching.

McKenzie's advice for athletes and others who engage in vigorous activity, and who have recently developed low back pain, is to try to expose the true cause of the problem. It is necessary to determine whether the pain appears *during* a particular activity or *afterwards*. If the pain appears during the activity, then the sport itself may be the cause of the problem.

To ascertain if low back pain is the result of slouched sitting after participating in a sport or other vigorous activity, observe your posture carefully and sit correctly, with the low back in moderate lordosis (curving towards the front), supported by a lumbar roll if necessary (*see* chapter two, page 16). This means *not* sinking into a 'comfortable' chair or slouching in a car after having played a few sets of tennis or a round of golf. It means sitting with meticulous attention to good posture (please review chapter two). Should pain occur following this careful attention to posture, then the cause is probably due to the sport in which you're involved, or the way you practise it. It would then be a good idea to have this looked into.

Behind the Wheel

Studies indicate that the incidence of low back injuries is on the increase, and experts point out that spinal problems can be induced by stresses incurred through lack of awareness of the spine's limitations. They suggest that many of these can be prevented through a better understanding of the structure and function of the spine (*see* chapter one) and of good body mechanics (*see* chapter two).

There are other measures motorists can take to protect their back and avoid needless suffering, inconvenience and expense. Here are some examples.

- Adjust the seat of your vehicle so that your legs can reach the pedals without being locked straight. Relax your knee joints.
- Sit as far back in your seat as you comfortably can, holding yourself naturally erect but not rigid. Relax your shoulders. Relax your jaw and breathe regularly.
- If necessary, support your back with a special back support, which some motor supplies stores sell; or try to obtain a lumbar roll (*see* chapter two, page 16). This prop will help protect your spine from the ill effects of side to side jostling when you drive over bumps or make turns.
- Don't clutch the steering-wheel like a weapon. This promotes tension. Hold it securely but in a relaxed manner.

Whether you're behind the wheel or are engaged in other activities, the way you hold and carry yourself, as well as the way you perform various movements, will affect the health of your back, and indeed your overall health. Many people experience pains and muscle spasms because they do not sit, stand, lie or work with their bodies properly aligned. When for example, we slouch at the wheel, we cramp organs and blood vessels. Our lungs can't expand fully and so the intake of oxygen, which is vital to body cells (particularly those of the brain) is inadequate. We begin to feel low in energy; we can't think clearly, concentrate properly or react spontaneously. We subject spinal muscles to greater than normal strain and promote aches and pain. With pain comes depression, and a vicious circle is created.

Here are further tips on posture:

- Sit on the 'sitting bones' (one under each buttock), rather than on the end of your spine. When not driving, try to rest your feet on a prop so that your knees are higher than your hips. This relaxes the back muscles.

- When walking to and from your vehicle, or elsewhere, develop the habit of walking tall to reduce stress. Tighten abdomen and buttocks so as to reduce the arch in the lower back. (The parts of the intervertebral discs within the spinal curves receive more pressure than those on the outside of the curves. They are therefore subjected to more wear and tear.) If you practise keeping your pelvis tilted somewhat backwards, it will reduce the lower back curve and help to prevent disc problems. Please review good posture in standing, Fig. 13 in chapter two, page 19.

- Stand as little as possible. In many non-industrialized societies, people generally stand only to move from one place to another. When they wish to chat, they squat (*see* Fig. 10, chapter two, page 14). Squatting reduces accentuated spinal curves, thus relieving stress on intervertebral discs, and gives back muscles a therapeutic stretch. There is a notable absence of back problems among people who habitually squat.

- Lorry (truck) drivers often take time off for a nap in their vehicles during long journeys. Other long-distance motorists lie down for half an hour or so when they begin to tire. Apply the squatting principle when lying: lie on your side; bend your hips and knees. Bring your lower knee closer to your chest than your upper knee. Arrange your arms for comfort. (*See* also Fig. 16, chapter two, page 22.)

- Avoid overweight. Excess weight places unnecessary strain on the spine and related structures. Review chapter three for information on nutrition. A rigid spine is more vulnerable to strains and injuries than a flexible one. Following are suggestions for some pleasant, easy-to-do little exercises you can try in a variety of places, such as at rest stops along the way.

- *Warm-ups.* Always warm up before exercising to avoid pulls and strains. Stand tall. Put your hands on your hips or stretch them sideways or in front of you. Inhale and rise onto your toes (hold on to a stable prop if you need to). Exhale and lower yourself to a squatting position. Inhale and come up to a standing position, on your toes. Repeat the up-and-down movement several times in succession, synchronizing breathing with movement. Rest. The warm-up is excellent for keeping the hip, knee and ankle joints flexible, to facilitate squatting. Practise the ankle, neck and shoulder warm-ups in chapter four, pages 50 to 54.

- Practise the *Posture Clasp* (Fig. 110, page 17) and the *Chest Expander* (Fig. 12, page 18) in chapter two.

- Practise the *Pelvic Tilt*, in any convenient position (see chapter five, pages 70 to 74).
- Use your breath as a resource during stressful times on the road. Inhale slowly, smoothly and deeply through your nostrils. Exhale through pouted lips, as if cooling a hot drink or whistling a tune. Repeat the exercise several times in smooth succession. Even slowing down your breathing, and making it smooth and deep can have a calming effect when you feel tension mounting as you drive. Remember to let go of tightness in your lips and jaw and to relax your other facial muscles.
- Using a seat belt with both chest and lap components gives protection to both the dorsal and lumbar spine. A properly designed headrest will give protection to the cervical spine.

Menstruation

Backache can occur both premenstrually and during the menstrual period itself. It is important to know if your backache is cyclic, or if it may be attributed to some other condition. If you have any doubt whatever that your backache is related to your menstrual cycle, you should have a general physical and pelvic examination by your doctor to exclude any medical or gynaecological disorder, such as fibroids or endometriosis, or medical condition such as lupus, which is dealt with later in this chapter on page 174.

Once it has been determined that your backache or back pain is a symptom of PMS (Premenstrual Syndrome) or dymenorrhoea (painful menstrual period), there are several things you can do to ease the discomfort. You can:

- Rest in bed in a position you find most comfortable (*see* chapter two, pages 21 to 22 for suggestions), with a heating pad or hot-water bottle, duly protected, applied to the affected part for short periods. (Sometimes local heat, used for prolonged periods, can increase pelvic congestion and therefore pain.)
- Try to practise a breathing or relaxation technique, such as those described in chapter eight. It is sometimes difficult to do this when you are in pain, but the effort is worthwhile. Tension and anxiety do increase pain (*see* chapter eight, page129 and 130). You might try the modified version of *Savasana* (page 143) and any of the breathing exercises described in chapter eight.

- Pay attention to your posture and carriage, as well as to your work habits. Good posture and body mechanics are important to backache prevention, as emphasized throughout the book. Please review chapter two (page 9 to 27).
- When not in pain, exercises to practise regularly for backache prevention include: *Squatting* (Fig. 10, chapter two, page 14); the *Lying Twist* (Fig. 24, page 54) and the *Cobra* (Fig. 65, page 82), both in chapter four; the *Cat Stretch series* (Pages 68 and 69), the *Pelvic Tilt* (Figs. 46 to 53), the *Bridge* (Fig. 54), the *Knee Presses* (Figs. 56 to 58), the *Star Posture* (Fig. 62), and *Pose of a Child* (Figs. 71 and 72) and its variation described in chapter seven; following the *Half Locust*, the *Spinal Twist* (Figs. 71 and 72), all to be found in chapter five; the *Single Leg Raise* (Fig. 93) and variations in chapter six, and the *Half Locust*.

Remember to warm up properly before practising these and other exercises. Please review chapter four.

Here are two other exercises you can add to your repertoire for helping to prevent or to relieve backache and back pain before and during your menstrual period.

The Legs-up Posture

In addition to being a useful adjunct to other pain-relief measures, this exercise is wonderful for relieving tired, aching legs and feet and for promoting all-over relaxation. Combine it with slow, rhythmical breathing.

1   Lie near a wall. Rest your legs against the wall so that they form about a 45° angle with the surface on which you are lying. Relax your arms at your sides, close your eyes and breathe regularly (Fig. 126).
2   Stay in this posture for several minutes.
3   When you are ready to get up do so, slowly and carefully: bring your knees towards your abdomen, roll onto your side and use your hands to help you into a sitting position (see Fig. 17, page 23).

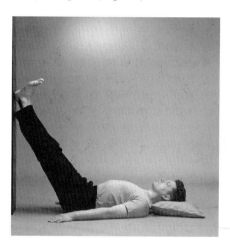

Fig. 126. The Legs-Up Posture

The Spread-leg Stretch

1 Sit naturally erect on your mat, with your legs stretched out in front of you and comfortably spread apart. Rest your palms on your legs (Fig. 127). Breathe regularly.

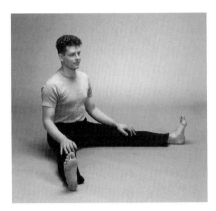

Fig. 127. The Spread-leg Stretch – start position

2 Exhale and bend forwards, at the hip joints rather than at the waist, sliding your hands down your legs (Fig. 128). Keep breathing regularly.
3 When you can bend no farther with absolute comfort, hold the posture for several seconds but continue to breathe regularly.

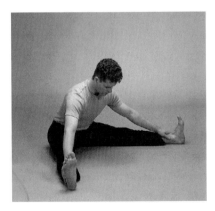

Fig. 128. The Spread-leg Stretch – bending forward from hips

4   Inhale and slowly come upwards again, to resume your starting position.

5   Place your hands on the mat beside you to help you into a folded-legs posture. Rest in this position or lie down and relax.

One other measure to try for back relief is a sitz bath. If you don't have a special sitz tub, improvise. Fill a large, deep basin with enough warm water so that when you sit in it your pelvis is submerged. (The water temperature should be between 38° and 46°C, that is, between 100° and 115°F.) Add more warm water to maintain this temperature, if necessary.

Ideally, your feet should not be in the water, which makes a basin more suitable than a bathtub.

Remain in the sitz bath for ten to 20 minutes and keep your upper body warm.

For more information on natural ways to overcome menstrual problems, read my book entitled *Pain-Free Periods* (*see* bibliography).

Pre- and Post-natal Back Chat

The not uncommon occurrence of backache in pregnancy is due, in part, to an altered centre of gravity and consequent increased lordosis (forward spinal curvature in the lumbar region), as well as to a relaxing of joints due to hormonal influences. There is also fatigue, which deters effort at maintaining good habits. Strict attention to good posture (*see* chapter two) is, however, of the utmost importance, to prevent strains, aches and pain. Keeping good abdominal muscle tone (*see* chapter six) is crucial as well for keeping back problems to a minimum both pre- and post-natally. The back exercises in chapter five are useful, with modifications where necessary, to suit your own situation. Remember to warm up adequately (*see* chapter four) before exercising.

Here are additional tips for pregnant women and those who have recently given birth:

- *Don't* wear high heels. It encourages poor posture. It aggravates the arch in your lower back and increases strain on spinal supports. Wearing high heels leads to a shortening of the hamstring muscles which, as mentioned in chapter one, page 7, are secondary back supports contributing to the tilt of the pelvis. High heels, moreover, put too much weight on the front part of the foot, and if the toes of the shoes are narrow, they make foot muscles rigid and tense. This, in turn, leads to tense leg muscles which cause tension of the back muscles.

- Tight stockings or tights are also bad for the back. They interfere with the relaxation of the toes and feet which, as just mentioned, have a bearing on how the back feels.

- Brassieres with narrow straps can cause aches in the shoulders and upper back, partly because of direct pressure and partly because of the rigid position into which they force the wearer. Both contribute to back tension.

- Make sure your work surfaces in the kitchen are of the right height for *you*: They should be about 5 to 8 cm (2 to 3 inches) lower than your elbows so that you don't have to stoop. Stand as close as you can to the work area and, if possible, rest your hips against it.

- When you must stand, try resting one foot on a low stool, a foot-rail or other prop about 10 to 14 cm (4 to 6 inches) above the floor (Fig. 129). This will relax the psoas muscle, which stretches from the lower back across the pelvis to the thigh, and relieve strain on the back.

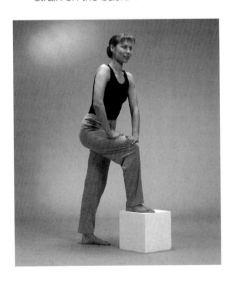

Fig. 129. Pre-natal exercise – standing one foot on prop

Caesarean section

Most women who have had a caesarean delivery are up and about the day after surgery. Early, graduated, consistent exercise is very important to the healing process and to promotes proper union of the incision edges. It is also essential to help to restore muscle tone and function of all body structures.

Since the abdominal muscles give reinforcement to the back (*see* chapter six), it is important that these be quickly strengthened through appropriate exercise. Start with a simple breathing technique. While lying comfortably, support your abdomen with your hands. Take a slow, smooth, deep breath in through your nostrils. Exhale steadily through your mouth while saying 'huh' or 'huff'.

Repeat this exercise several times in succession. Don't be afraid that your stitches will pop; they won't.

Progress to simple leg exercises. From a supine position, with the small of your back firmly pressed to the surface on which you are lying, and with your legs stretched out in front (Fig. 130), slide one heel towards you (Fig. 131), then away from you, several times in slow succession. Repeat the exercise with the other leg. Remember to keep breathing regularly.

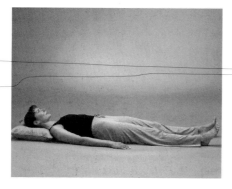

Fig. 130. Post-natal – supine, legs stretched out

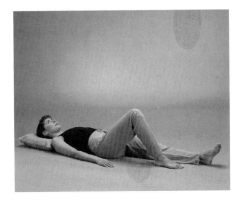

Fig. 131. Post-natal – heel towards bottom

As your strength and energy return, work slowly up to the exercises in chapters five, six and seven. Always warm up first (*see* chapter four). Also recommended is the practice of breathing exercises and some form of meditation every day. Suggestions are given in chapter eight.

For more in-depth information on keeping fit during and after pregnancy, you may wish to look at my book entitled *Easy Pregnancy with Yoga* (*see* bibliography).

Relieving a Tired Back

There are several conditions that cause sufferers to feel low in energy generally and to experience back fatigue not infrequently. The first that comes to mind is ME (myalgic encephalomyelitis), also referred to as CFS (chronic fatigue syndrome). This is a condition in which normal body and central nervous system functions have been disturbed and deranged. There are two schools of thought as to the causes: one is that of persistent viral infection due to non-effectiveness of normal immune mechanism; the other is that persisting viral infection triggers an abnormal immune response. Whatever the cause or causes of ME are, fatigue is one of the most frequent symptoms.

SLE (systemic lupus erythematosus, or 'lupus') is another disorder that tends to curtail activity. Lupus is sometimes classified as an auto-immune disease, in which the body turns in on itself, as it were. It is also described as a collagen disease. Collagen is the cement-like material that holds body cells together (*see* chapter one). Anything affecting the integrity of the body's collagen will cause it to weaken. People with lupus often report persisting aches and pains in joints of the back and elsewhere, and they tend to tire easily.

Yet another debilitating condition is MS (multiple sclerosis), a chronic progressive nervous system disease of unknown cause. Many people with MS function seemingly normally, but as the disease advances, energy is affected and mobility restricted.

As we age we tend to feel fatigue more readily than when we were younger. Also, we may not be as mobile or active. Often the back is the first place where we feel the symptoms of ageing.

Fatigue is a warning symptom. It signals that the body is tired and should be rested. To ignore this warning is to court trouble in the form of pain or injury. When your back is tired, you need to rest it. It's that simple. You will find the lying positions described in chapter two (Figs. 15 and 16, pages 21 and 22), the *Pose of a Child* (Figs. 71 and 72, chapter five, page 85), and its variation in chapter seven (Figs. 78 and 79, page 86) useful. You could also sit in a recliner (easy chair) that provides good support for your spine, arms and legs. While resting, practise a breathing or relaxation exercise such as described in chapters four and eight.

To strengthen the back, and the abdomen which gives reinforcement to the back muscles, practise the basic version of the exercises in chapters five and six, making sure that you warm up properly, as suggested in chapter four. Keep your legs well toned by practising the exercises in chapter seven. Shortened hamstring muscles increase the arch of the lower back, thus imposing strain on back structures.

If you find some of the exercises too challenging for you, then omit them, or modify them to suit your particular state. The neck, shoulder and ankle warm-ups in chapter four are easy to do and help to prevent tension from building up. The *Pelvic Tilt* and the *Knee Presses* (chapter five, pages 71 to 73 and 77 to 78) are not difficult. The *Single Leg Raise* (chapter six, page 106) and the *Butterfly* (chapter seven, pages 112 and 113) are also among the easier exercises you might wish to try.

Sex Without Back Pain

There are few illnesses that should be allowed to interfere totally with physical intimacy between two loving partners. Even if you don't feel well enough to engage in sexual intercourse, simply holding each other close can be a wonderful experience.

Various illnesses, such as those mentioned in the previous section, cause the sufferers to tire easily. They may produce stiffness and aching joints. They may cause pain. Even the fear of pain will decrease interest in sex: fear generates tension and tension can eventually produce pain.

People being treated with the drug cortisone tend to bruise easily and some develop painful hips. Cortisone also produces sexual apathy in some individuals. The bruising or fear of bruising may inhibit the desire for sex or make the other partner feel guilty about causing injury. One partner may sense the other's need for gratification but, feeling exhausted, is unable to meet this need. The other partner may feel denied or rejected.

In any case where there are factors that have the potential to damage sexual relationships, it is vitally important that the partners at least attempt to understand each other's feelings. It is essential that apprehensions, fears, feelings of guilt, etc. be sensitively discussed. Don't hesitate to seek professional help, if necessary. Reduced sexual ardour need not mean lack of love or interest, but this should be made clear.

Keep communication lines open. Make adjustments. Show consideration. Remember: having a chronic illness or growing older does not necessarily mean that sexual activity must be curtailed or eliminated.

Postural adjustments

Couples who have a warm, loving relationship will find ways over or around sexual obstacles. Orgasm, in fact, is said to trigger a release of natural cortisone, which can be helpful in reducing pain. (Cortisone is a hormone produced by the cortex, or outer portion, of the adrenal glands which are located above the kidneys).

If your problem is facet joint strain, you are probably better off lying on your back, with your partner on top. If pain strikes during intercourse, try gentle pelvic tilting (*see* Fig. 47, page 70) to reduce the curve in your lower back and diminish strain on the joints.

The pelvic thrusting movements of sexual intercourse may work as a mobilizing exercise when you lie supine. These are reminiscent of the *Pelvic Tilt* (Fig. 47, page 70). Your knees should be bent and your feet placed flat on the bed or wherever you are lying. If you assume an 'all-fours' position, with your partner behind you, the pelvic rocking movements are similar to the *Cat Stretch* (Fig. 44, page 69). Be careful not to accentuate the concave arch of the back. The 'all-fours' position is also worth a try if you like lying on your back but your partner is much heavier than you.

Another position for women to try is one reminiscent of the *Knee Press, Variation II* (*see* chapter five, Fig. 58, page 78), omitting step 4 of the instructions and keeping your head flat. The partner kneels, and the woman is thus spared the weight of the man's body. She can support her bent legs or her partner can. A little experimentation and creativity will quickly teach both partners the best arrangement for them.

If you have back problems, try lying side by side, arranging your limbs for maximum comfort.

A man with back pain may be more comfortable sitting in a chair than lying down. The female partner can then sit astride him and be the more active participant. Here, too, the pelvic tilting exercises come in handy.

The following is a little exercise which, although not involving the back muscles, is useful for women to practise regularly. It tones up the perineum, which is the lowest part of the torso, between the legs, thus improving support for pelvic organs.

Breathe regularly. On an exhalation, tighten your vagina and anus. Hold the tightness until your exhalation is complete. Inhale and relax. Repeat the exercise once now and again later.

You can do this perineal exercise almost anywhere because no one can see what you are doing. You can do it during sex to enhance your partner's pleasure.

Other exercises to practise regularly to keep you fit for sex include: the *Lying Twist* (Fig. 24, page 54), the *Cat Stretch* series (Figs. 42 to 45, pages 68 to 69), the *Butterfly* (Figs. 97 and 98, pages 112 to 113) and the *Spread-Leg Stretch* described in this chapter on page 169.

Modify any or all of these exercises to suit your particular situation.

Check local libraries and bookstores for books about fostering mutually satisfying sexual relationships. Some are specially written for people with mobility difficulties. All emphasize the importance of good communication through talking, listening, touching and other forms of tenderness. Also check community services for leaflets on this subject.

Backup

Tips for self-care and for preventing back pain

Doctors and other health professionals emphasize personal responsibility in caring for your back. They stress the importance of putting good postural habits into daily practice, and of exercising faithfully in order to control back problems so that those problems don't control you.

The background information presented in this book, along with exercise instructions and illustrations will provide you with basic resources for looking after your back with intelligence. The additional hints to follow will supplement the information given in preceding chapters.

* If you feel a back spasm coming, lie on the floor, with a cushion under your head and buttocks for support, and rest your legs on a chair. Position your buttocks as far under the chair as possible so that your trunk is at right angles to your thighs.

* If you hurt your back, apply an ice pack to the sore area for about 15 minutes every four to six hours. This will anaesthetize the affected part, minimize inflammation and pain and prevent further swelling.
* If your back becomes stiff, try heat. A heating pad or hot-water bottle (properly covered) applied to the stiff area, or taking a hot bath or shower will bring some relief.
* Massage is often wonderful for a sore back. It helps increase blood flow to the hurting area, relax the muscles and decrease pain.
* When muscles or joints are inflamed and painful, they must be adequately rested to ease discomfort and permit healing.
* Avoid crossing your legs. It tilts the pelvis too far forwards and increases lordosis (spinal curve convex towards the front, as at the small of the back). This puts strain on the back. Whenever you sit on a chair try to have your knees level with, or slightly higher, than your hips.
* If you must read in bed, sit upright and place a pillow under your knees to counteract strain of the lower back. If you read lying down, the strain on your neck can lead to degenerative changes in the cervical spine (pertaining to the neck), and to arthritis and pain.

- Carry a baby as close as possible to your body or against your shoulder.
- Don't bend over to make a bed. Rest one bent knee on the bed, if you can, and brace yourself with your hand to ease pressure on your back.
- Support your abdomen with your hands when you cough or sneeze.
- Don't overload your briefcase.
- Keep luggage to a minimum and make it lightweight. Buy luggage with shoulder-straps.
- Find ways to exercise during the course of your day's work: deliver memos from office to office whenever you can; walk up and down stairs instead of using the lift (elevator); park your car well away from your destination so that you have to walk. The exercise will burn up excess fat tissue, improve blood circulation and muscle tone and maintain good mobility. All these are essential to a healthy spine.
- Squat to put away papers in filing cabinets or to retrieve them (*see* Fig. 10, page 14). Do not bend over.
- **Remember the five back basics: regular exercise; proper body mechanics** (*see* pages 9 to 27); **adequate rest; good nutrition and weight control, and effective stress management.**

Glossary

Anaesthetize
Make insensible to pain.

Analgesic
A remedy that relieves pain.

Antacid
An agent that neutralizes acidity, especially in the digestive tract.

Antioxidant
An agent that prevents or inhibits oxidation (process of a substance combining with oxygen).

Articulation
The place of union between two or more bones; a joint.

Cervical
Pertaining to the region of the neck.

Collagen
A fibrous insoluble protein found in connective tissue, including bone, ligaments and cartilage.

Cyclic

Periodic; occurring in cycles.

Disc

See Intervertebral disc.

Dorsal

Pertaining to the back.

End plate

A layer of cartilage covering the upper and lower surfaces of intervertebral discs.

Endocrine glands

Glands whose secretions (hormones) flow directly into the blood and are circulated to all parts of the body.

Enzyme

A complex protein that is capable of inducing chemical changes in other substances without being changed itself.

Epidemiologic

Pertaining to the study of epidemics (appearance of a condition or infectious disease that attacks many people at the same time in the same geographical area).

Facets

Bony surfaces of the rear part of a vertebra which match up with similar surfaces on the neighbouring vertebrae and guide their movements.

Facet joints

Joints formed by vertebral facets (*see* above).

Gynaecologic

Pertaining to the study of diseases peculiar to women.

Hamstrings

Three muscles on the back of the thigh. They flex the leg and adduct (bring toward the midline) and extend the thigh.

Immune
Protected against disease.

Immune response
The reaction of the body to substances that are foreign or interpreted as foreign.

Intervertebral disc
Broad, flattened disc of fibrocartilage between the bodies of vertebrae.

Kyphosis
Refers to a spinal curve that is convex towards the rear.

Lordosis
Refers to a spinal curve that is convex toward the front. The normal curve of the lumbar region of the spine is lordotic.

Lymph
An alkaline fluid found in lymphatic vessels.

Matrix (bone)
The intercellular substance from which bone develops.

Orthopaedic
Prevention or correction of deformities, especially of the body's bony frameowork.

Osteoporosis
Porous bone. A disease characterized by low bone mass and structural deterioration of bone tissue.

Prone
Lying horizontal with the face downward. Opposite of supine.

Pulses
Edible seeds of leguminous plants, such as beans, lentils and peas. Also known as legumes.

Quadriceps
A large muscle on the front of the thigh.

Respiration
The act of breathing; inhaling and exhaling.

Sacral
Pertaining to the sacrum, a triangular bone located at the back of the pelvis. It is made up of five fused vertebrae.

Sacroiliac joints
The joints formed by the hip bones and the sacrum.

Skeletal
Pertaining to the body's bony framework.

Spondylolisthesis
A forward slipping of the lower lumbar vertebrae on the sacrum.

Spondylolysis
The breaking down of a vertebral structure.

Supine
Lying on the back, with the face upward. Opposite of prone.

Synthesize
Uniting elements to produce compounds. The process of building up.

Thoracic
Pertaining to the chest.

Torque
A force producing rotary motion.

Vertebra (pl. vertebrae)
Any one of the 33 bones forming the spinal column.

Vertebral column
Spine or spinal column. Backbone.

Viscera
Organs enclosed within a cavity, especially the abdominal organs.

Bibliography

Abraham, Edward A., MD, *Freedom from Back Pain. An Orthopedist's Self-Help Guide*, Emmaus, Pennsylvania: Rodale Press, 1986.

Airola, Paavo, Ph.D., *Dr Airola's Handbook of Natural Healing. How to Get Well*, Phoenix, Arizona, Health Plus Publishers, 1974.

Aladjem, Henrietta, *Understanding Lupus: What it is. How to treat it. How to cope with it*, New York: Charles Scribner's Sons, 1982.

Atkinson, Holly, MD, *Women and Fatigue*, New York: G. P. Putnam's Sons, 1985.

Barnard, Neal, MD, *Foods That Fight Pain*, New York: Harmony Books, 1998.

Benson, Herbert, *The Relaxation Response*, New York: William Morrow, 1975.

Black, Joyce M., MSN, RNC, and Matassarin-Jacobs, Esther, Ph.D., RN, OCN *Luckmann and Sorensen's Medical-Surgical Nursing* (4th ed.) Philadelphia: W. B. Saunders, 1993.

Brena, Steven F., MD, *Yoga and Medicine*, Baltimore, Maryland: Penguin Books, 1973.

Cailliet, Rene, MD, *Low Back Pain Syndrome* (3rd ed.), Philadelphia: F. A. Davis Company, 1981.

Caruth, Fran and Thompson, Flora, *Transfer and Lifting Techniques for Extended Care*, Vancouver, Canada: 'Transfer Manual', P.O. Box 1341, Postal Station A, 1983.

Colbin, Annemarie, MA, CHES *Food and Our Bones*, New York: Penguin Putnam, 1998.

Corbin, Dr Charles B., and Lindsey, Dr Ruth, *Concepts of Physical Fitness with Laboratories* (7th ed,), Dubuque, Iowa: Wm. C. Brown Publishers, 1991.

Davis, Adelle, *Let's Eat Right to Keep Fit*, New York: New American Library, 1970.

Deyo, Richard A., MD, MPH, 'Fads in the Treatment of Low Back Pain' *The New England Journal of Medicine, Vol. 325*, No. 14, Oct. 3, 1991, pp. 1039-1040.

Faelton, Sharon, and the Editors of *Prevention Magazine*, *The Complete Book of Minerals for Health*, Emmaus, Pennsylvania: Rodale Press, 1981.

Fardon, David F., MD, *Osteoporosis: Your Head Start on the Prevention and Treatment of Brittle Bones*, New York: Macmillan, 1985.

Fahrni, W. Harry, MD, FRCS (Edinburgh), M.Ch. Orth. (Liverpool), *Backache Relieved Through New Concepts of Posture*, Springfield, Ill.: Charles C. Thomas, 1966.

Fine, Judylaine, *Conquering Back Pain. A Comprehensive Guide*, New York: Prentice Hall Press, 1987.

Fromm, Erich, *The Art of Loving*, New York: Bantam Books, 1963.

Gaby, Alan R., MD *Preventing and Reversing Osteoporosis*, Rocklin, California: Prinia Publishing, 1994.

Gulledge, A, Dale, MD (Guest Ed.), 'Depression and Chronic Fatigue', *Primary Care. Clinics in Office Practice*, Vol. 18, No. 2, June 1991, Philadelphia: W. B. Saunders, 1991.

Hall, Hamilton, MD, *The Back Doctor*, Toronto: McClelland and Stewart-Bantam, 1980.

Hausman, Patricia, MD, *The Calcium Bible*, New York: Rawson Associates, 1985.

Hewitt, James, *The Complete Yoga Book*, New York: Schocken Books, 1977.

Hittleman, Richard, *Yoga: The 8 Steps to Health and Peace*, New York: Bantam Books, 1976.

Imrie, Dr David, and Barbuto, Dr Lu, *The Back Power Program*, Toronto: Stoddart Publishing, 1988.

Kaufmann, Klaus, *Silica. The Forgotten Nutrient*, Burnaby, Canada: Alive Books, 1990.

Kounovsky, Nicholas, *The Joy of Feeling Fit*, London: Pelham Books, 1971.

Kraus, Hans, MD, *Backache, Stress and Tension*, New York: Simon and Schuster, 1965.

Lagerwerff, Ellen B., and Perlroth, Karen A., *Mensendieck Your Posture and Your Pains*, New York: Anchor Press/Doubleday, 1973.

Lauersen, Niels H., MD, and Stukane, Eileen, *PMS. Premenstrual Syndrome and You*, New York: Pinnacle Books, 1983.

Leboyer, Federick, *Birth Without Violence*, New York: Alfred A. Knopf, 1976.

Liang, Matthew H., MD (Guest Ed.), 'Musculoskeletal Pain Syndromes', *Primary Care. Clinics in Office Practice*, Vol 15. No. 4, Dec. 1988. Philadephia: W.B. Saunders, 1988.

Livingston, Michael, MD, *Beyond Backache. A Personal Guide to Back and Neck Pain Relief*, San Diego, California: Libra Publishers, 1988.

McCaffrey, Margo, RN, MS, FAAN, and Beebe, Alexandra, RN, MS, OCN, *Pain: Clinical Manual For Nursing Practice*, St Louis: The C. V. Mosby Company, 1989.

McKenzie Robin, FNZSP, DIP, MT, *Treat Your Own Back* (4th ed.), Waikanae, New Zealand: Spinal Publications Ltd, 1988.

Mindell, Earl, *Earl Mindell's Vitamin Bible*, New York: Warner Books, 1979.

Mindell, Earl, *Earl Mindell's Pill Bible*, New York: Bantam Books, 1984.

Natow, Annette, and Heslin, Jo-Ann, *Nutrition for the Prime of Your Life*, New York: McGraw-Hill, 1983.

Nicolas, James A., and Hershman, Elliott B. (Eds). *The Lower Extremity and Spine in Sports Medicine*, Vol. 2, St Louis: C.V. Mosby, 1986.

Noble, Elizabeth, RPT, *Essential Exercises for the Childbearing Year*, Boston: Houghton Mifflin, 1976.

Pelletier, Kenneth R., *Mind as Healer, Mind as Slayer* New York: Dell Publishing, 1977.

Phillips, Robert H., Ph. D., *Coping With Lupus*, Wayne, New Jersey: Avery Publishing, 1984.

Schatz, Mary Pullig, MD, *Back Care Basics*, Berkeley, California: Rodmell Press, 1992.

Schneider, Dr Johannes, 'Silica. A vital element for good health'. *Alive Canadian Journal of Health & Nutrition*, No. 80, pp.13-15.

Shreeve, Caroline, M., MD, *The Alternative Dictionary of Symptoms and Cures*, London: Century Hutchinson, 1986.

Stanton, Rosemary, *Eating for Peak Performance*, Sydney: Allen & Unwin, 1988.

Stroebel, Charles F., MD, *QR The Quieting Reflex*, New York: Berkley Books, 1983.

Tanner, John, MB, BS, MSc, *Beating Back Pain. A Practical Self-Help Guide to Prevention and Treatment*, Toronto: Macmillan of Canada, 1988.

Tessman, Jack R., *My Back Doesn't Hurt Anymore*, New York: Quick Fox, 1980.

Turner, Roger Newman, BAc, ND, DO, MRO, *Banish Back Pain. Effective self-help with the aid of simple home remedies*, Wellingborough, England: Thorsons Publishers, 1989.

Van Straten, ND, DO, *The Complete Natural-Health Consultant*, New York: Prentice—Hall Press, 1987.

Weller, Stella, *Easy Pregnancy with Yoga*, London: Thorsons, 1999.

Weller, Stella, *Pain-free Periods*, London: Thorsons, 1986.

Weller, Stella, *Yoga Therapy*, London: Thorsons, 1995.

Weller, Stella, *Yoga for Long Life*, London: Thorsons, 1997.

Weller, Stella, *The Breath Book*, London: Thorsons, 1999.

Weller, Stella, *Well Being for Women*, New Alresford, England: Godsfield Press, and New York: Sterling, 1999.

White, Augustus A. III, MD, *Your Aching Back. A Doctor's Guide to Relief*, New York: Bantam Books, 1983.

Woolf, Anthony D., MD, MRCP, and Dixon, Allan St John, MD, FRCP, *Osteoporosis: A Clinical Guide*, Philadelphia: J. B. Lippincott, 1988.

Workers' Compensation Board of British Columbia, *Back Talk. An Owner's Manual for Backs*, British Columbia, Canada: Workers' Compensation Board of Canada, 1987.

Yogendra, Sitadevi, Smt, *Yoga Simplified for Women*, Santa Cruz. Bombay: The Yoga Institute, 1972.

index